The COLOR DIET

by Dick Chudnow

Illustrations by Roger Huebner
Additional Material by Karen Kolberg

outskirts
press

THE COLOR DIET
"One color a day keeps the doctor away."

*This book is dedicated to our Son, Nick, who was the sweetest,
funniest person I've ever known*

Quotes From Foodies

Mahatma Gandhi, *Fashionista: I will not begin to eat until my nation is in the buffet line.*

Buddha, Figure Head, Writer: *I said "yummmmmmmm" I don't know how it turned into "ommmmmmmm."*

Mohammed: Author, God: *"I will kill you, and take the food you are chewing out of your infidel mouth".*

Moses: Tour guide: *"I saw a burning bush, honest I did. I saw it, it was burning and everything. Here, have another piece of flat, tasteless bread".*

Judas Iscariot, Disciple: *"Darn, I didn't find the Seder Afikomen again. Mark got 20 shekels for it. This is the last supper I go to at Mrs. Christ's house".*

Julia Child, Author, Wine Taster : *"Cooking without wine is like going to prom with your cousin, starting the opera* with *the fat lady singing, or like playing hop scotch without the scotch."*

Anthony Bourdain, Author, TV celebrity, Eater: *"Food is a great way to start off any meal".*

Nick Castle, Director, Musician, and "The Shape" *"A tasty dinner is like a good meal, only the same".*

Table of Contents

Acknowledgements

I'd like to thank everyone who bought this book, those who are thinking about buying it, or those who are just thumbing through it at the checkout line, while waiting for their husband, wife, partner, or au pair, with whom they are having an affair, to unload the groceries from the shopping cart onto the conveyer belt.

We would also like to thank the small bookstore manager (5' in mukluks), Martin (not real name. I mean 'Martin" is a real name, a lot of people have it, but it's not Ed Miliskus's real name), who is a very supportive fellow in the writing community, and stocks many books written by local authors.

We need to thank this miracle of society, because this institution, God love it, has convinced its followers that if you have more than 2% body fat, and aren't thin, famous, thin, rich and thin, you should not go out in public.

A big *je vous remerge* to Peter Roget for his famous dictionary of synonyms: *Roget's thesaurus.* Did you know that he dated Emily Bronte, and was thinking of calling his book the Brontethesaurus". I think that is an astonishing, astounding, awesome, conspicuous, eye-opening, fabulous, fascinating, impressive, inspiring, marvelous, phenomenal, portentous, prodigious, remarkable, staggering, stunning, stupendous, sublime, surprising, wonderful, and wondrous fact.

What about 'ol Betty "Crock-pot" Crocker and her tablecloth plaid cookbook. Calories hadn't been invented yet, but I know that my Mom's book was loaded with them. Lick the cover and you'd gain a pound from the ingredients caked on after the years of use.

A big shout out to my wife, Jennifer Rupp. "HEYYYYYY, JENNIFER RUPP!!" Jennifer, under the pen name, Jennifer Trethewey, is an actual published writer of Scottish romance novels. She critiqued the book for me and made some valuable suggestions - like: "What about fishing for a hobby?"

Also, thank you to the multi-talented Roger "Hubba Hubba" Huebner, who did the illustrations for the book. Roger was also the sound effects performer for ComedySportz Milwaukee, and once made a life-sized Styrofoam chicken, pepperoni pizza, and Zamboni that we used in our shows.

Fourthly or fifthly, thank you to the bulti-talented Karen Kolberg™, one of the originators of ComedySportz. Karen helped edit the book and contributed most, if not all, of the cornier humor, because, she, like most humans, consists of about 60% water, but unlike most humans the other 40% is pure corn.

Lastly, thank you to my Grandma Sarah Chudnow, whose amazing recipes would have been handed down from generation to generation, had any of them been written down. It probably wouldn't have mattered anyway, because they would have had instructions like: "a little flour, some salt, maybe a couple of eggs, I don't remember, Anyway, if you have to write the ingredients down, you shouldn't be baking anything. " My Grandma thought measuring tools were for sissies.

I often wondered why she wasn't wasting away because at dinners she wouldn't come to the table to actually eat any of her incredible food.

Here's a typical dinner scene: (Names haven't been changed, because there's not chance any of my relatives would ever read this book)

SCENE: GRANDMA AND GRANDPA'S HOUSE, DINING ROOM

AUNTS AND UNCLES AROUND THE TABLE

ABE: Ma! Sit and eat with us!

GRANDMA: I will, I will. Move the potatoes so I can set down another bowl of schmaltz for Sammy. Sammy loves schmaltz.*

SAMMY: Come on, Ma, sit, eat.

GRANDMA: Who wants more gribbenas (fried chicken skins)? Bennela, you don't like the brisket?

BEN: Ma, I had sixteen pieces already. Sit with us!

GRANDMA: I will, I will....

FINALLY, UNCLE ERV AND UNCLE JOE TACKLE GRANDMA, WRESTLE HER INTO A CHAIR, HOLD HER DOWN, AND BEGIN SPOON FEEDING HER.

GRANDMA: The liver! The liver!

ABE: You sit, Ruthie will bring it in from the kitchen.

GRANDMA: I didn't make liver. You're sitting on mine!

AND........SCENE.

*Schmaltz is like lard, only 500 more times deadlier. Allow me to analogize: If lard is a swimming pool, schmaltz is the Atlantic Ocean. If lard is a firecracker, schmaltz is an atomic bomb. If lard is the playground bully, schmaltz is Andre The Giant.

Acknowledgemints

A huge thank you to my packs of Listerine Breath Strips™, and the Tic Tacs™ I always keep in my car. You know, in that little compartment under the radio? Nothing else really fits in there. Also, a big debt of gratitude to my good buddy, knew him since high school, Al Toid. *

*The above was contributed by Karen Kolberg. The Color Diet Institute doesn't necessarily support, nor is responsible for, and expressly disclaims all liability for damages of any kind arising out of the reading of the above chapter, and does not constitute an endorsement by the Color Diet Institute, or their products and/or their services.

Disclaimer

Let's make something perfectly clear, clear as legally allowed, as clear as Big Cedar Lake back in the 1950's before Jet Skis™ were invented.

Here at the CDI™, our purpose is not to talk you into losing weight. Our goal is simply to present the true, generally agreed upon, solid facts about food and how it should be bought, prepared, and eaten. We not only don't care if you are "overweight," in fact, we don't even recognize that word. We have friends who are "bigger than life", but we don't see them as "fat". We don't laugh behind, or in front of their backs.

We are not meglophobiacs*. In more fact, we are not at all judgmental about anything. We don't see people as old or young, tall or short, male or female, handsome or ugly, white or black, roly or poly, smart or dumb, lost or found, naughty or nice, Marianne or Ginger. We truly believe that every and all body formats are all part of nature, and God's plan. If a person is ok with their body type and weight, then everything is jake with us.

This book is intended to help those who have lost faith in diets and diet books. But let's not think of this as a "diet book". Let us think of it as…oh, how do you say it….ah….a" true miracle". We are fed up to here (our third chins) with all the diet book authors out there who *don't* believe all body types are OK, jerks, yes I said "jerks" who believe that washboard abs and hourglass figures are the only acceptable body types.

Boldly, we say, please, go ahead, have 100% body fat. If you are "healthy" and can do a roundabout on the parallel bars, then we could give an otter's nipple about your body and the shape it is in.

*Megalophobia is "the morbid and irrational fear of large or oversized objects". Look it up.

Our Guarantee

If, on the other hand, losing weight is your goal, we are so confident in this diet, that if you do not lose weight, if you don't look better, smell better, don't have sex at least twice a day, and you are unable to do the splits, there is a chance we might return most of the money you spent on this book.*

We will also give you the telephone number of a smart as a whip ** lawyer who might be happy to sue us for the entire amount minus shipping, handling, and 54¢ a mile.

That written, we are proud to say that almost every single time we have been sued, we have won. We almost lost once, but the judge ended up throwing the case out of court. Here's the true story, and if it isn't true, then may whatever gods or avatars you believe in strike me down with sores. Here's that not made up story:

A slovenly man, a husband of a woman who was on the Color Diet, upon bad advice from a shady lawyer not on our preferred lawyer list, decided to sue us. It seems, according to courtroom artist renderings, his wife started using the Color Diet and lost 75 pounds in two months. She became so svelte, and so desirable, she left her husband for a wealthy slum landlord. Of course the husband lost the case because not only was he a complete snot-gobbler, but also because the ruling judge had lost 30 pounds on the Color Diet.

ADDENDUMB: We regret having to report that the ex-husband became a broken, lonely man, living in a cold water flat in Boise, where his only food source was the Mormon Church's leek and cucumber haggis. Sad story, true, But....there is a happy ending.

We sent this ex-hubby a free copy of the Color Diet, and now he is a microbiology engineer for Hertz, and lives in a gated community in Boca Raton. Not only that, he and the judge in the case now live together, and plan to get married as soon as it is legal in Florida, which may be after both are dead, but they do have plans for a funeral/wedding ceremony just in case.

*The amount we might return to you depends on how long you kept the book and what kind of shape it is in. If we can resell it, we'll return the full amount. But, none-the-less, if you were dissatisfied with any part of the book, excluding the content, the cover, the font, or the incomprehensible sentence structure, before you get any dinero, we will first send you a new copy of the book. That's right, an entire new copy of the book you just hated free of charge.

But we think, honestly, and with all sincerity available, if you are dissatisfied with the program, double negatives be damned, you probably can't lose weight no matter what you do or don't do. If you carefully follow the instructions in the book, there is no chance in heaven, hell, or wherever you think you go when you die, of you not being a better you.

SIDEBAR: That written, if you must sue us you have to follow these easy steps:
1. Send in four partially clothed pictures of yourself from all four sides of your pre-body, and four of your post-body.
2. You should be wearing the same clothes in both sets of pictures, and your facial expression must be the same in both sets.

3. The pictures must be taken in front of a notary who then must sign the two sets of pictures.

4. You must swear, in a real court of law, in front of a real judge, not a television judge, like Judy, Milan, or any of the other 30 or 40 TV judges, on a stack of Color Diet Books, that you really did not lose weight.

Or.....

Just call and leave us a message stating that you didn't like the book. The call must be under 400 words, and have two references to Civil War Southern generals. One of our helpful, pigeon English speaking assistants will be glad to try and help you with your claim. If that doesn't work for you, let us know, and we will switch our operations to an undisclosed location somewhere in Mumbai.

**Whips, in a triple blind study have been proven to be the smartest non-human objects this or any other universe, scoring over 750 on their credit reports.

Prologue

Definition: In favor of a chunk of wood.*

* Kolberg again.

THE "D" WORD

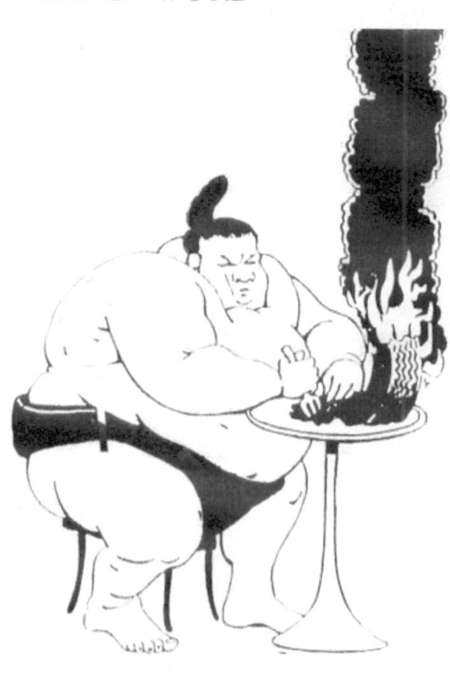

Before I delve into the Color Diet itself, and the details/specifics/ of the ECT/F (Enzymatic Color Theory/ Fact) let's talk about what we mean/understand by the word/expression "diet". Diet is a word that we are hearing plenty/a lot of lately. It's a word often bandied/bantered about by charlatans and or politicians/ con artists who should be forced to eat burning rubber tires with a Styrofoam fork.

So, what does the word actually mean?

Webster says: "diet (di'et) n. The legislature of certain countries such as Japan. So what's all the fuss? Except for Sumo wrestlers, how many fat Japanese people do you see in a day? We don't think one has to be a High Beta Frappe to get the point.

Health vs/ Beauty

My parents used to give me a lot of advice. For instance: "The most important thing is that you have your health." Later they would add: "…and if you don't have that, at least have good health insurance coverage because pre-existing conditions will bankrupt you like they did Uncle Schlomo." They would also tell me that "family is the most important thing." I had to ask: "Wait, you said health is the most important thing. Which is it? Family or health? Or is it "family-health? It didn't really matter because what your parents are actually thinking when they give you all that advice is: "Please don't do anything to embarrass us," and who can argue with that kind of logic?

Roly-poly children embarrass their parents, even if the parents are whale-like themselves. Now, as opposed to Biblical times, when husky was all the rage, people believe that good health is useless if you look like a poorly stuffed mattress. That is a sad fact, one in which I don't condone, and take a knee when the "be skinny" flag is flying.

Furthermore, in this day and age, unfortunately, we are told that the only thing that matters in life is that we look good to others. If you look in any fashion magazine, something I wholeheartedly do not recommend, you see pretend people who are moonlighting as pipe cleaners. These magazines scream at us: "Beefy is bad, gaunt is good!" They, the dark side, want to make us feel that being a blimpish butterball is worse than anything you could be, including a burglar, a cradle-robber, or a lawyer. They went you to see fat as an ugly malignant, evil, festering putrefaction. They quote that best seller, the Bible: "Aaron was as to the fatted calf." They, the thinsters, go on to say that chunkiness stands between you and looking good to others, like a movie studio guard stands between the public and the main gate at Paramount, where you can't get in unless you know movie stars, writer, and directors like I do, or if you re wearing a tool belt, and/or carrying a clipboard. By the way, these aforementioned directors, writer, and movie stars, with the help of my diet have lost over a combined 5,000 pounds.

And, by another way, the film-flamists say that the term "big-boned" is just an excuse that the corpulent use to keep eating whatever and whenever they want. But dietologists are just now revealing that there is such a thing as having big bones. A security guard who works for the TSA told me that he may x-ray 500 people a day, and of that 500, over 25% have big bones.

Also, we realize that even though a person's bones may be huge, the stuff that grows around those ones is just as big. It's not like the bones go all the way to the skin, that would be, in scientific terms, weird. So, yeah, your bones might be big, but so are the cushions that surround the bones. Ergo, ipso facto, adoindictum, fat is merely an illusion that doesn't exist, so relax

Living The Lie

"You know what?"

"What?"

"Big butt, that's what."

Mickey Pierson, grade school friend.

Grade school inanities aside, it's OK to live in the "I'm a perfect weight for my height fat and sassy land, or to wallow in misery in your "big boned dream world." You have a lot of company. But why agonize?

I know I used to compare myself to people who were bulkier than me. "I don't eat deep fried butter at the fair like that woman. "I don't need a triple X-wheel chair like *that* guy. " "I don't shop at Omar's Tent Bizarre like *that* person. But one day I was in a carnival fun house, and the reflection in the convex mirror (the one that makes you look skinny) was of a hefty, yet devastatingly handsome man and I was standing right next to him, looking enormous. Did I care? I was taught to, so yeah, I thought I should do something about it.

So I took the quiz in *EAT MAGAZINE*"

The quiz:

1. Do you have to have someone tie your shoes for you because you can't bend over?

2. Do you need a mirror to find your genitals?

That's as far as I got. It was enough for me to further my research to find something that would help me lose weight, tie my shoes, locate my genitals, and still be able to eat all the food I wanted to eat.

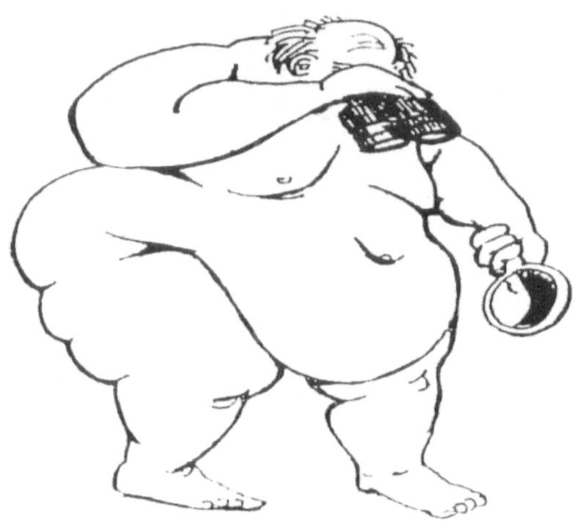

Why Another Diet Book?

Actually, in all honesty, or a goodly portion of it anyway, writing a book was the furthest thing from my mind. Even further than watching a Medea movie, riding the Tower of Terror rollercoaster again, or texting the Pope. Writing a book was right up there on my bucket list of things to never do, because basically, according to a Cosmopolitan quiz, I'm functionally illiterate. ("Functionally illiterate" is sort of being like "legally blind," which is awful, but still better than being "illegally blind.")

The sad fact is that most of my teachers in parent/teacher conferences would say things like: "Have you thought about trade school for Richard? Or: "you know, Mr. And Mrs Chudnow, they are doing wonders with electroshock therapy these days."

I was large for my age, but then again, I was large for any age, and therefore an easy target for classmates. Often, after school, Leon Pirkans, who was the only third grader with a girlfriend, would poke me in the stomach and say things like "When's the baby due Dickie?" I'd put on my brave face and say: "Sticks and stones may…" But before I could finish, Leon would break a stick over my head and shove me to the ground, and then his girlfriend would bonk me on the head with a stone,and roll me around like a whiskey barrel.

People can be cruel. Some intentionally, others unintentionally.

My own mother once told me: "you're not so fat honey, Aunt Tully is *fat*. One morning I woke up to a sign that looked hastily painted on the side of our house: "Chudnow, your not fat, you're just 3 feet too short."

The worst insult, though, was from one of the therapists my parents sent me to. "Richard," she said, "remember, it's what's on the inside that counts, and perhaps in your case, it's seven banana cream pies." Tears streaming down my face, I bolted from her office. She ran after me yelling: "Richard! I'm sorry! I didn't mean it! I meant three or four *pieces* of banana cream pie! *PIECES!*"

Fast forward decades. I was semi-retired (I used to drive a large truck*) I had already tried almost every diet out there, and found that none of them worked for me. But now I had some free time. I had to decide what to do with it. I could have taken up a sport, but I've heard that when you play sports, you sweat. That was not for me. Stamp collecting? No, not stamp collecting, I didn't get many letters. I also thought about continuing my education and going back to school, but I realized I would look ridiculous carrying a backpack though the halls of a junior high.

Then it hit me like a bolt from the blue, or like a punch to the gut, or like when my brother taught me how to play: "Who Can Hit The Other Softer" and made me go first.

I could help other people!

I could help people from having to go through the same kind of bullying *I* went through. I would be giving back to the world.

Now writing this book made total sense to me. But, before I put finger to the keyboard, I needed to do some research.

I got down to business and looked up every diet book and diet in Wikidietpedia, consulted diet gurus, health practitioners, and even sent a letter to my idol, Rachel Rae. I asked if she would be willing to write an introduction to my book. Her agent wrote back saying: "Rachel would rather have a Taco Bell bean and beef chili bowl enema than write anything for your idiotic book." I thought that was a little harsh, but didn't reply because Rachel is too darn cute to hate.

Undeterred, I kept up my diligent research. I went to the local library, which was closed*, so I went to the book store where I browsed through all of the diet books I found, and learned that most of the diets said pretty much the same kinds of things.

"NO CARBS! NO FAT! NO SUGAR! NO SALT! STOP BEING SO FAT!. None of it rang true. None of it spoke to me, Or if it did, it was in a bossy, snide, know-it-all voice.

The bullies were back, and my suspicions were confirmed. All these books and diets were scams written by people who just wanted to make a buck off morons like me who at one time bought into society's obsession with thinosity.

These books were partially baked scams written by con artists. Their diets were conceived by pen people who wrote diets with cockamamie, cobbled together recipes. I am sure that maybe some of the authors were sincere in their misguided beliefs, but some were obvious bull-twaddeling tricksters, heinous scammers of such magnitude they and their schemes couldn't be described by using words in the English language alone. You would need the Spanish: "Estfa, the Yiddish: "Ganif, The Swedish: "Svindel, and the Southern: "Skayam".

In any language, these diets are simply fakes of a fraud of a con. Mere hocus-pocus-hanky-panky. Ruses, nay, deceptive ploys, and devious dodges, hoodwinking flimflam. Sure, we are fooled by the authors' jacket cover photos, and the fact that they contribute to Indian schools, and generally fight for justice and truth and the American way, but peel away all that really honorable stuff, and what you find are foodie Barnums, shady double dealing fast-talking dupers, who defraud poor pigeon pushovers like sitting ducks in line for a ride on the sucker express.

"Sham" is the only word, besides all the other ones I looked up, that can suitably describe what these diets are. And you know what you get when you add an E" to "sham"? Yes. "SHAME". Shame on you, you purveyors of fakeness.

*I think libraries should be open 24-7 like hospitals, airports, jails, and Waffle Houses.

Sham Diets

THE BEVERLY HILLS DIET::

The Beverly Hills Diet was the first fad diet. It come out in 1981, years before humans had perfected the fad diet. Back then it was just called a "diet." The "fad" part came years later with the full-blown diet craze. Before 1981 no one really gave much of a skinny. Big boned? Wear a muumuu. "Fat"? Wear a girdle. Yes, you had your Jack Laanne, but that was pretty much it as far as diet plans were concerned. We smoked, we gorged, and danced the hootchie coo. The Beverly Hills Diet was at first meant only for people living in Beverly Hills, and specifically, Beverly Hillians who lived north of Olympic Boulevard.

In the Beverly Hills Diet, the dieter must only eat in restaurants, preferably five star restaurants, on Rodeo Drive. They all must be restaurants at which Beverly Hills Diet creator, Judy Mazel has eaten. The food must also be eaten in a certain order.* The salad, then the dessert, the entree, then finally the beverages. Stray from that order and Judy herself will descend upon your table, and will acid reflux your out of order butt until you tofu the line so to speak.

*Unless the diners are my Mom's friends, then the order is:

SCENE: RESTAURANT BAYSIDE WISCONSIN

WAITER: May I help you?

SYLVIA: Darling, do you have real challah? You know, the twist?

WAITER: I'm sorry we just have white, rye, and whole wheat.

SYLVIA: Oh. Ok, then….let me…oh…how about….(SILENCE)…. what about…...(TA DA!) an English muffin. You have English muffins?

WAITER: I will find one. I may have to run home and bring one back, but you will *have* your English muffin.

SYLVIA: You are *funny!* Are you married darling? Because Lillian has a daughter, who's cute as a button and smart! She went to Bryn Mawr.

LILLIAN: Culver Junior College, with honors.

SYLVIA: Whatever, she might be interested in a good- looking man with a job and a sense of humor.

LILLIAN: I'm sure he has a girlfriend himself. Do you? Do you have a girlfriend, sweetie?

WAITER: I'm gay.

EVELYN: SLAPS HIS ARM That's what I thought! Nothing wrong with it I think everybody is gay now a days.

WAITER: Yes, probably. Can I get you something ma'am?

EVELYN: I'll have an order of rye bread, toasted on one side, with margarine, or non-salted butter. You don't remember because you are, what? 20? 25? But back in the day, oleo was outlawed in Wisconsin. We'd have to sneak it over state lines.

SYLVIA: I remember that! You felt like a criminal for God's sake.

WAITER: Will you be having a salad?

LILLIAN: I think (STUDYING THE MENU).......the ah....
Caesar....no...Cobb...no....just make it a house salad with dressing
on half of it. What kind of dressing do you have boobela?

WAITER: Ranch, Italian, Thousand Island, vinaigrette, Russian, garlic
avocado, Caesar, honey mustard, French, and Miracle Whip.

SYLVIA: Miracle Whip? Why? Miracle Whip tastes like something
that came out of a boil.

ALL LAUGH

SYLVIA: I'll have the Thousand Island, but make it 900 Islands, I'm
on a diet.

THEY ALL SCREAM WITH LAUGHTER

WAITER: Ok, I think I've got it, Anything else.

SYLVIA: I think we're good sweetie.

LILLIAN, That's it for me darling.

EVELYN: I'm not eating, I have a procedure at 4.

WAITER WALKS OFF

LILLIAN: SHOUTING. TOOTSIE! CAN I HAVE A SIDE OF
HUMMUS TO GO PLEASE? Or no, never mind, David can't eat
that. NEVER MIND HONEY! (TO THE GIRLS) Piles.

THE GRAPEFRUIT DIET: "Ruining lives since 1980"

This diet is mainly for people who don't mind malnutrition.
Grapefruit supposedly has magical powers of digestion. Grapefruit is

98% acid, but not the fun kind. No daily recommended amount of grapefruit acid. has been established by the Nutritional Acid Institute of America. This diet may have been created by employees of the Grapefruit Industry. There's a "catch" to the Grapefruit diet. The catch is that we have found out that grapefruit, because of the toxic acids found in it, can negate the positive benefits of medications, cause severe impotence, blet, impede a person's ability to see, hear, or smell, and or make people unsympathetic to less fortunate people who can't afford Jimmy Chong purses. Other than that, it may help you lose weight.

THE SOUTH BEACH DIET

The South Beach Diet dictates the you eat seasoned shells, sand, and sometimes sautéed globs of tar that have washed up on the shore from one of the numerous oil spills that were so popular in the 90's. The authors of this diet proclaim that tar and sand are prodigious emetics. Even if you eat other food, you'll be throwing up most of the time, therefore not getting any calories at all. The shells themselves are rich in calcium, so there's that. But the sad fact is that if you get too much sun, and then you tend to come up with bad ideas. Like wind-surfing.

THE CARBO LOAD DIET

In the Carbo Load, you eat lots of carbs. You eat all the carbs you can get your grubby mouth on. All the carbs at home, at work, and on the way home. You can eat all the carbs the ""NO CARB DIET" diet people don't eat.

THE PRITIKIN DIET

Pritikin was the absolute Barnum of diet "gurus", which may be the reason he was shot. Just sayin'. Pritikin advocates ingesting whole grains, fruits and vegetables, almonds, flaxseeds, and other legumes. Isn't that nuts? I like fruits and vegetables as much as the other guy, but I also like porterhouse steak grilled in butter, smothered in butter marinated mushrooms, with a side of butter, slathered in mash potatoes.

If you ask me to give all that up, I don't care how much I weigh. I hope I don't have a heart attack or die in any way, but if I do, I hope it's after I finish my steak.

THE ATKINS DIET

The Atkins is the exact opposite of the Pritikin, and spelled differently, only Atkins might still be alive. Nobody knows. Not really. I've done the research. Anyway, Atkins wants to take away the stuff Pritikin wants you to eat. Chet Atkins, Robert's cousin, claims that the diet helped him in his country-western music career.

In this diet, you don't eat carbs. Ever. How insane is that? Why don't you just wear a chasity belt, never shop for clothes, or just scoop your eyes out with a soup spoon. We think that this diet was a parody of other diets, but hardly anyone got the joke. But, and that's a big but, it proved to be a mega-hit.

I can have my steak on the Atkins, but not my jelly-filled donut, or the dark chocolate cake I order after I porterhoused. Look, I maybe have five, seven years left, I'm not going to deny myself anything. But let's say I wasn't so very close to the beyond, would I eat the same things I do now? You bet your chickpea compote I would.

The story between these two wackadoodles, Atkins, and Pritikin is interesting. It reminds me of the beautiful poem, "Jack Sprat" by Gertrude Goose, the English author and accomplished maypole dancer.

It goes something like this: "Jack Spratt could eat no cheese, so Mrs. Spratt said: "I'll have that please." This was the basic argument between the two diet giants of our day. These two megalomaniacs despised each other and their opposite ends of the diet plan spectrum. In Wikidietpedia, you can read about the history of their food feud. I read it and it reminded me of the Tesla-Edison feud. Furthermore, I think, and this is just me, if one were to analogize, Tesla would be Pritikin, and Edison would side with Atkins. Or vice versa, that's not the point. The point is something else. The "else" eludes me right now. I think it had something to do with the Rachel Rae, "How to Be Adorable While Cooking Food" diet. As a spinoff of the Atkins, there is a "No Carb Diet, which has become popular amongst people who basically want to tell their friends: "I'm on the no carb diet."

THE DIET DIET

Not a complex plan. The simplicity of the Diet Diet Plan is: Don't eat as much as you usually eat.

RACHEL RAE'S "BIG ORANGE BOOK"

The "big R" wants to acquaint the dieter with "food with a sense of humor". I'd say she achieves her purpose. Her recipes, while not using anything toxic, are hysterical. Rachel is a woman after my own gut, which is from whence one laughs.

She's also developed "Yum-O" a charitable foundation dedicated to helping parents and children develop a healthy relationship with food. I sincerely think that is pure genius. RaeRae, as Rachel likes me to call her (she calls me "That Nut") recommends that to establish the relationship between the food and self, children should get to know their food before they eat it. Rachel recommends that they take their food on play dates, chat with it, buy it gifts, invite it to family functions, and maybe get into couples therapy with a qualified psychiatrist. Rachel, kookily cute.

THE DESPERATE HOUSEWIVES COOKBOOK

Another celebrity cook, recipe, and diet book. These mostly sad women are pro-oxidants, as opposed to the antioxidants.

What I find especially interesting in this book is that one of the authors is Bree Van de Camp. *Brie Van de Camp?* Here are some of her recipes:

Brie and Beans Salad Fraiche.

Soft Cheese and Pork Fried Bean ala frozen fish sticks

Fried Beans and Little Sausages In A Hot Cheese Fondu.

Cheese and beans. It sounds like an euphemism for the swears when you hit your thumb with a hammer. "Cheese and beans that hurt!!!

THE VEGETARIAN DIET

My big brother, Larry Chudnow, used to say: I know some vegetarians, they are mostly people, but I wouldn't want to eat with them, because I've found that they are as bright as the animals they don't eat. But then again, my brother used to say: "A riddle, a riddle I suppose. What has two cheeks, but not a nose?" (I didn't get it until I was 12)

THE TUMMY TUCK DIET

In this medieval procedure, usually done on an autopsy table, you are gutted like a pig, your stomach is folded over like a soft taco, then stapled together. It may or may not help you lose weight. Your tummy is smaller so you may feel fuller faster, but when did feeling full ever stop us from eating more?

WARNING: Be careful of getting the hiccups, because there is a good chance your staples might pop.

THE PAPERCLIP DIET

This diet is exactly the same as the Tummy Tuck Diet, only much much cheaper.

LIPOSUCTION

In this procedure, someone, sometimes a doctor, sucks the fat out of your body with a long, sharp vacuum tube, and replaces the fat with protein bars. The people who perform this obscene practice used to do abortions in French opium dens.

THE GHANDI DIET

Sit. Meditate. Don't eat until some improbable task is completed. Like licking your own elbow, or sneezing with your eyes open, or holding one's breath until the Electoral College is abolished.

THE RICHARD SIMMONS CRAZY AS A RABID HYENA ON METH DIET

Jump around like Jerry Lewis in his early films, and then wait for the spaceship.

What was so disturbing with each one of these diets Was that you had to give up something, or in some cases, *everything* you like to eat. Why should you have to give those things up if you don't know what fate has in store for you? Who knows what could happen? You could walk out of your front door and get hit by a cement truck, or flattened by a rogue comet, or be the victim of a random pit bull attack.*

Personally, I don't want to be the guy, who is on his way to heaven or "h" "e" double hockey sticks, who thinks: "Man! Had I known that my neighbor was a homicidal maniac, I would have eaten the last chocolate eclair!"

But did I really want to go deeper into this whole diet "cabal"? If I really wanted to blow the whistle on the diet conspiracy, I had to think deeply about it, which is not easy for me without hemorrhaging, so I knew I had to go spelunking. I always spelunk when I need to think. Who doesn't? I went to my favorite cave.

*Pit bulls have been unjustly stereotyped on TV judge shows. Defendants argue their innocence with statements like: "My pit bull is a very loving animal and extremely gentle with my kids." (SHOWS PICTURES OF KIDS LYING ON THE PIT BULL). My pit would never attack the mailman like defendant said he did! She was playing with him when the mailman stuck his leg in my pit's mouth. And those three Jehovah Witnesses? They brought it on themselves.

Diet, A History

My spelunking was going well, and I was thinking very deeply indeed, when a huge rat, or small dog, or possibly Chucky from the movie of the same name, scurried up my pants leg.

I screamed like a little girl and ran.

The first rule of spelunking is "never talk about spelunking". The second rule is "Never run in a cave." I've already violated rule #1, as for #2, when something has run up your leg in a cave, rules go out the window. Sprinting, I went head first into either a stalagmite or a stalactite, staggered backward, and fell into a pit. I was uninjured, and when I looked up, I saw that my flashlight shone on some crude scratches on the cave wall.

I climbed over some stalactites, and under some stalagmites, or vice versa, and found that the writing continued along the entire wall. Runes? Cunioform? Gangs? I took a bunch of pictures crawled to the exit, and drove, poste haste (I speak fluent Latin), to the one hour photo booth. The guy said they'd be ready in an hour, I wisecracked (I also speak fluent wisecrack), that I never would have known had he not reminded me that I was at a "one hour photo booth". He said:

"Now it'll be an hour and fifteen minutes". I shut my yap, and got some coffee. When they were done, I rushed them to my spelunking partner (one should never really go spelunking alone, many spelunkers have ended up in magical pirate scenarios from which they never return), Deeters "The Gentle Giant, " Stormbulski. Deeters works in the local ancient history cave artifact center franchise, which is located in the basement of Boswell books on Downer Avenue. Ya know, On Mwaukees's fashionable East Side? Down by the Starbucks across the street from the new parking ramp?

Deeters was busy but when I told him what I had found, he agreed to take a look. He put down the papers he was studying (which looked like some kind of research comparing the ancient pyramids with to-day's pyramid schemes). With a wry smirk ("Wry Smirk" would be a great name for a band or improv group) that said "Ok, I'll check out your little 'pictures' for you. Let's look at your 'monsters in the closet.'"

I wasn't sure why he did air quotes when he said "pictures" and "monsters in the closet", but Deeters is air quoting all the time. He's like the air quote "king".

He looked, cleared his throat, hocked in a bucket he kept by his desk, and got out his "InterpreScope" to accurately translate the drawings I had found. His smirk quickly fell from his face. He picked it up from the floor, put it in his breast pocket, then climbed the ladder to get a huge tome (redundant) down from a book shelf. He swept all his junk off the table opened the book, and began checking the photos against some scribblings in the book.

Turns out that it was a book of ancient manuscripts. It took him about a minute or so, maybe 90 seconds, minute and a half, or a little less, or a little more, I'm not sure, my memory isn't clear on how long it took him. Let's say as long as it took me to write how long it took, until he gasped, and sat bolt upright. I had never seen Deeters so excited. I could tell he was excited because his eyebrows stood straight out, and his hearing aids flew out of his ears.

Deeter told me that the "markings" were over 40,000 years old, and very valuable. "You are a very rich man, my friend'" he said. I told him that money does not concern me. All the reward I need is knowing that I have made a contribution to society, that I did my part as a "human being" on a planet we all share, and a Maserati.

The writings described some rituals of the tribe. One wall depicted a virgin who was about to become a sacrifice to the gods. It explained in great detail how she saved herself moments before being shoved over the cliff, by having sex with the shaman. The story ended with probably the oldest, and worst joke ever told. When the shaman was asked if he would still execute her even though he had been intimate with her, he replied: "execute her? I hardly know her."

There were also explanations of dating rituals of the time. Contrary to popular beliefs, a cave man did not just walk up behind a cave woman, knock her out, and drag her back to his cave. There was some foreplay involved. There were gentle taps to the head in the courtship period, and before the woman could be beaned and dragged away, the man had to go to her parents and show them the size of his club, then, and only then would he be able to haul her away. The couple would then find a cave of their own to raise their hairy families. The married women stayed at home and never participated in the hunts like the single women did. Instead, like women thought the ages, they made sure that the delivery guy was out of the cave by 5:00

The rest of the writings were what interested me the most. It turned out they were a sort of diet book. The writings explained that in early days, before they had fire, knives, forks and/or napkins, they would just sneak up on a sleeping animal, or one that was in the midst of sexual congress, take a bite and run. They could kill smaller animals like sabertooth rabbits, sabertooth prairie dogs, and even ate of the fleshy saber-toothed trout. (A animals in those primitive days were saber-toothed).

Deeter read me one recipe for "Saber Toothed Otter"

And I quote:

"Ingredients: one otter.

Instructions:

1. Catch otter.

2. Kill otter.

3. Remove saber teeth.

4. Eat otter.

5. Put otter teeth on necklace for Valentine's Day.

Then, little Deeter (Deeter, contrary to his nickname, is barely two feet tall) told me that according to the inscriptions, these mostly human people, who didn't even read at a second grade level, had a shaman in their midst. The word "shaman" evidently was a term for the one in the tribe who would "shame" them into doing his will, This shaman noticed that fat tribes had vanished. He surmised that the animals targeted larger tribesmen for their meat. The recipes in the book were written to keep the tribespeople from getting too fat, and thus becoming targets for the larger saber-toothed animals. This tribe eventually evolved into the species of humans called "personal trainers."

The Scoop On Fat

Let's look into this so called "Fat," shall we? Let's do. Fat is an important foodstuff for many forms of life, and fats serve both structural and metabolic functions. Fats are a necessary part of one's diet, but, what exactly are they? Where can they be found? Why are they called "fats"? What are the implications? Once we answers those questions, and only after we answer them, will we know. Not before we answer them. After.

We have already established that being corpulent has been looked upon as something to be avoided at all costs. This is true across all social, political, psychological, and mythological aspects of our society. We should ask ourselves: "How did this happen? Who's behind this glorification of thin?

Choose one or more of the following:
1 The fashion Industry
2. Pharmaceuticals
3. Hollywood
4. The media
5. You
6. Me

The correct answers are 1 through 5.

But wait! There's more! Many bulkologists, through thousands of intricate, complex, sophisticated research projects, over a period of many days, which were funded by my inheritance, have discovered things that are too complicated for the average person to understand.

Fat Spectrum

The same scientists, who have asked to remain nameless, have disclosed that they have found a whole spectrum of fat out there, of which we are just now becoming aware. They go on to say that when it comes to fat, there is a dark, underground. They continue this alarming news by telling us that they can state this unequivocally because they have their own "deep esophagus" informant who told them that there is actually the equivalent of an "Area 52" of fat, and that it is carefully guarded by the U.S. Army and Marine Corps. And just as UFOs are most likely stored in hangars in Area 52, so are the kinds of fat they are talking about stored in U-Haul-like lockers in our own hidden government's secret compounds. They concluded by telling me that they're pretty sure "the fat is out there."

"So what?" you ask. I agree. It sounded too alarmist to be true to me. It sounded like the warnings they give you in some lead-ins to the 11:00 news:

"Are school lunches killing your child? (They are) one woman's story at 11." "Can looking at yourself in the mirror cause mental health problems? (It can) News at 11." "Are video games a Russian plot to steal our kids? (They are) You should hear what this ex-KGB secret agent told us. News at 11."

I had to ask: Is fat really that bad for us? Maybe there is a "soft side" to this despised excoriated, natural resource. I hate to get all scientific all over you, but if you look up the definition of "fat" in the dictionary * this is what you will find:

"Fat, having superfluous flesh."

The key word here is "superfluous." There are negative connotations surrounding the word "superfluous." I disagree with the negative meaning of the word. Pimples are superfluous, body lice are superfluous, hemorrhoids are superfluous, liver spots are superfluous. No one wants an extra nostril, another thumb, a third armpit, or two belly buttons. I think that any one of those would Make you somewhat of a curiosity, and maybe a freak to less enlightened people, including your mother, who, as a mother, is supposed to love all her children, even your brother, who may, as of today, or may not, still be in jail for animal abuse.

The "F" word has become the epitome of vileness, with some negative words like:

"Fat chance": "Very little or no chance."
"Fatuous": "Foolish or inane."
"Fat-al": "Resulting in death."
"Fat-igue": "The condition of being very tired.

But let's take a step back and look at fat from another angle, perhaps through a microscope.

You know that grade school lesson where they put a drop of drinking water under a microscope and revealed a whole nation of little amoeba-like things swimming around? Well, when you put a droplet of fat under the same microscope, there aren't armies of squiggly things swimming around. None.

Ergo ipso facto dereguire: Fat may be healthier for you than you drinking water!

And remember, about a paragraph or two ago when I gave you some of the negative definitions of fat? Well, let me tell you, Billy Jo Bob-tail Cat, there are other more modern-day even smarter, more cunning linguists that have other meaning of the "F"word.

"Fat of the land": "The good part."
"Phat": " Indonesian for 'good'"

"Fat-herland": Your home.
"Fat-hom: "To understand."

Going back to Webster, we find this: "Fat, solids that are esters of glycerol and certain fatty acids. Present in some plants and in the adipose tissue of animals, forming a reserve energy source." Did you read that? "Forming a reserve energy source." So there you go, it's not a bad thing to have a "reserve energy source." To quote ex-con Martha Stewart: "It's a good thing."

Definitions aside, be that as it may, most things considered, the term "fat" really shouldn't be a generic term. Why?

Because there are so many different kinds, and types of this so-called "fat".

Most of the forms and types of fat in the spectrum are good for you. So we have to ask: "Do we really know exactly what fat is? Is it really superfluous? Or…instead, is it simply a "super-fluid!"

*The dictionary was written by Noah Webster, not Daniel, a cousin. Daniel invented the sneaker. Noah was not related to the ark builder.

TYPES OF FAT

Following is a list of fats in the fat spectrum. I've included where you can find them, what they look like, and what their functions are. Once again, keep in mind, that not all of these fats are bad for you, that is, IF, and as you can see, that's a big "if", you follow the Color Diet™

Name: SKIN FOAM
Layer: Epidermal
Location: Evenly dispersed.
Type: Small layer of water depleted fat. Like indoor/outdoor carpet.

Density: Firm fat, only 10% water.

Attributes: This is the best kind of fat to have. This is a partial store of energy. Good for speed walking, swimming laps, and shopping sprees.

BABY FAT

Layer: Subdermal (not so cutaneous)

Location: Abdomen, breasts, ankles.

Derivation: Formed at birth, or when someone asks if your pregnant, and you're not.

Density: Puffy fat, like the grease at the bottom of a pan in which bacon was made.

Attributes: This type of fat gives you a soft, pliable, likable appearance. It is good for corporate board meetings, first dates, and psychiatrists.

GLANDULAR FAT

Layer: Cutaneous.

Location: Neck, knees, underarms and eyes.

Type: "Sappy Fat." Runs from glands like tree sap.

Density: Composition of melted generic lard.

Attributes: Keeps the glands from drying up. Rich in lipids, it gives your lips that fullness that is so acceptable now-a-days.

CELLULITE

Layer: Retro-cutaneal

Location: Thighs, triceps and knuckles.

Derivation: Springy, bumpy, like unmixed concrete.

Density: 50-50. Spongy. Like a bath sponge, and 50% nutty putty.

Attributes: This type of fat has been the most maligned. But it is, in fact, the only kind of fat that keeps your bones safe. It is a healthy cushion for vulnerable spots on your body. Like the term indicates, it also complements the cells in your body. It is an ex-cell-lent source of energy.

DEMI DERMAL PASTE

Layer: Metadermal.

Location: Buttocks and possibly ear lobes, but mainly buttocks.

Derivation: Mucusy, runny, snot-like. Like when your infant has a bad cold.

Density: Oozy fat, 70% gel.

Attributes: Dermal Paste is mostly for the aesthetic of the entire inner body. If you could open a body and take a little look-see, you would find that people with this type of fat have the shiniest, sleekest, most aero-dynamic organs of any human.

TURBO BLUBBER

Layer: Megadermal

Location: Ev ree where.

Derivation: In the brains and tissues of walruses and Wild Asian Water Buffalos.

Density: 100% pure. No additives. Sometimes it's call "virgin fat".

Once you have built up this kind of fat in your system, it is very difficult to get rid of even if you wanted to. However, I must say that it is the kind of fat that is richest in reserve energy. It is the best kind to have if you are a survivor of a shipwreck and are going to be stranded on the water for weeks, months or years with no food except an occasional flounder, or raft mate. The kind of fat you find on reality shows.

Enzymatic Theory

All this talk about fat behooves me to talk about enzymes. Enzymes are key to the Color Diet Theory.

You might be thinking: "Enzymes, I can't think of anything I'd like to talk about less, other than the Sex Crazed Housewives of Racine". Yeah, who cares about enzymes. You think whatever you want, because this in America the land of the free for God's sake, and we can think or believe anything we want as long as we hear it on Fox News or see it on Facebook.

But I'll say this: If you think enzymes are not important, you are a wrong thinker. You are in denial. I thumb my nose at you and your pathetic ignorance. I would go on to say that your nonchalance about something as incredibly important as enzymes makes you a gob-mouthed, beef-witted, snivel twitted, canker-blossomed clot-pole.

I kid. I kid. Those insults don't apply to you, they were just fun to write.

The important of enzymes is obvious to both the casual (you) observer, and the professional (me) observer because "Enzyme" is one of the few words in the English language that finds a "zy" combination in a word that isn't a Czechoslovakian name.

Furthermore, if you break down the word you'll find that "en" is short for "end," and the suffix, "cyme," has its roots in the Latin: "zyma" which translates somehow, (which we won't go into now because you don't need to speak Latin to do the Color Diet) into "Acid" So thus, we have "end acid." In Ancient Rome, they used to use enzymes for out of body experiences, like we use our LSD today.

Scientists have learned, though the grapevine that all enzymes are proteins, but not all proteins are enzymes in every instance. Think about that for a second.....what did you think? Yes, me too.

Those same scientists, in different off-white smocks, have discovered that all proteins are probably enzymes too, and that proteins are the building blocks of all living organisms. Humans, animals, plants, and microorganisms are all made up of proteins. Even proteins are made up of proteins. Every part of the human body is built of proteins. Proteins constitute about 80% of the dry weight of muscle, 70% of the dry weight of skin, and 90% of the wet weight of blood.

Some other scientists, not the ones who thought that enzymes are definitely proteins, found that like all other proteins, enzymes are made of amino acids, and each enzyme is made up of between a hundred and up to a million amino acids placed like pearls on string. Each amino acid is bonded to the next by chemical bonds each having its own unique sequence of... blah blah blah.

All you need to know, are these important facts: (you know that they are important because they are in bold, and italicized in size 16 bold Bodoni Oldstlyle Italics)

Fact: Food color is determined by enzymes
Fact: The stomach can digest only one color enzyme a day.
Fact: The mixing of these enzymes is what causes weight gain.
  Our stomachs can deal with only one enzyme at a time.
  One day. One enzyme

Why is this the case? Here's what happens when you try and digest two enzymes in one day:

The naturally colored Enzymes (one produced by nature, not in a laboratory) get confused, addled, and if you are a crossword nut, then you could say they are "at sea." You could also say: "bolloxed" if it were a real word. They are like Moses in the desert, like Ronald Reagan in his last two years of his second term, or like my Uncle Mac who didn't forget how to pee, but forgot what a toilet looked like.

If there are two enzymes in the stomach at the same time, the digestive juices don't know which color (enzyme) to attack, so they give up and go back to their digestive nests, or "enzidiums" and the food in your stomach is left undigested. Undigested food has nowhere to go. After sitting there for a while, they turn into fat cells through the process of "Endomytosizing."

There is an equation known by most enzymologists:

FAT = UNDIGESTED DOOD, AND CONVERSELY, UNDIGESTED FOOD = FAT.

Fat has been outed. Enzymes are out of the closet! So let's talk about the specific enzymes involved in the fascinating world of Enzymmation.

MEET THE ENZYMES:

RED: Di-lithy-oxymeta-carbolosate

GREEN: Oxymeta-lithyl-carbolododo GxD

WHITE: Carbo-doodoo-0xyclean deitilylru-lol

ORANGE: Meta-mucil-carbolosate2xY@K

BROWN: DI-LITHIUM-baglunch-Vm#2

YELLOW: Sulfa-urathanate 1/2-2P

PURPLE: Npl.

There you have it! The COLOR DIET theory!

Now that you are familiar with the technical/scientific ins and outs of diet, fat, and enzymes, let's put all that mumbo jumbo, jibber-jabber- tongue gaggle into a clearer, more concise, understandable kind of jargon even *I* would understand. Let's find out how all those complex formulas fit in with a successful diet plan.

What Do Genes Have To Do With It?

I have over heard, at various social functions, people saying that genes play a part in being overweight. Yeah right. Genes. Huh! What are they good for? Absolutely nuttin'. They may not even exist. What? No genes?? Am I saying that the Earth is flat? That the moon landing was faked? Maybe I am. Maybe the moon landing was "one step for man, one giant bunch of hooey for mankind. First in moon-landings, last in healthcare!" When newscasters, hot shot reporters, and other town criers announced that astro-men landed on the moon, I wasn't fooled. I mean look at Star Wars, and other movies that look even more believable than the footage of the moon landing. Right, the best they could do was "live" footage of some shadowy square-headed, bulky suited monster walking in slo-motion? I've seen power point demonstrations clearer and more believable than that.

But people are easily fooled. Look at Barnum, Einstein, Houdini, or Dr. Phil. Tricksters all. The gullibles, as I like to call them, are the same sophisticates who see some pictures of swirly, long things, they call Dinosaurr Nuclear Acid or something like that and think: "Wow, that is fantastic! What will be next? Secret brain juices? The cure for chilblains? Who really did the crop circles? These are the same human-like people who buy into anything they see on TV or read in the USA Today. These are the people who bought "Blu-Blocker" sun glasses, "My Pillows, and/or wear tin foil hats to block alien control rays (which didn't work, by the way). If there were a book about these people it would be called Gullible's Travels."

Now, I'm not saying that gene theory is a bunch of hooey, not at all. I'm writing it. Do you know how small a camera would have to be to get into a human cell? Smaller than the teeniest, tiniest camera makers could ever make. But, despite the mocking cries of "ooof-poof, twiddle-twaddle, and horse-pucky, the debate goes on.

In total, and unneeded fairness, one can ask: "Ok, if there actually are these genetic thingys, which I think we have adequately proved false, some questions still need to be begged.. So please, we beg you, let's ask the difficult questions.

1. Is "gene" just the name of the guy who perpetrated the scam? Is he the same guy who made the machine that Joe Joe made go, and that Art Art blew apart?
2. If "genes" are a thing, can some people be born without them?
3. Can someone have too many "genes"?
4. Where do "genes" go when we die?
5. How many calories are in one gene?
6. What is a "gene pool"? Can "genes" swim? Are they like sperm?
7. When you lose weight, do you also lose "genes"?
8. Can a doctor surgically add or take away "genes"?
9. Do animals have "genes" too?

These are all questions that have probably been debated for centuries, maybe more. Maybe less. Nobody knows. No one may ever know. No one may ever care.

Being the opticalmist (I see goodness in the future), I think we will find the answers. It may take years, but surely if there is a future, either here on Earth, or some other more advanced planet, answers will abound. Maybe it will be a planet where there are no questions. Just answers. But for now it's a never ending cycle of questions and answers, questions and answers, on into infinite foreverness, so don't think about it, because it's depressing.

Finally, you have to admit that people who believe this genetic hooey are not very bright. In fact, they are so dumb that once they tried to put their M&M's in alphabetical order. They think that Eartha Kitt was a set of garden tools. When they saw a sign at the movies that read: Under 17 Not Admitted", they went out and got 16 friends.

When they heard that 90% of accidents happen at home, they moved. At the bottom of the application where it says "sign here," they wrote "Libra." I heard that when they missed the #44 bus they took the #22 bus twice. They are so dumb that when they saw the sign on the freeway that said: "Airport Left", they turned around and went home. Once they sat on the TV and watched the couch. Rumor has it that when they looked in the lake, and saw a reflection of themselves, they jumped in and tried to save themselves from drowning.

I kid. I kid. I respect all people. No matter how moronic they are. Again, I kid. But they do have to call information to find the number for 911.

The Color Diet

Now that I have gotten the prescription for a healthy life in The Color Diet:

Rx:"A color a day keeps the doctor away",

I want to make sure it is successful for you. Diet gurus may have their particular theory, but they all agree that there are five ingredients for success.

Here are those five ingredients:

ONE: A SAFE, NUTRITIONAL MIX

Our bodies, being bodies, and working as bodies do, are really very complex engines, and from years, maybe months of studies devoted to just how these precision instruments work, we've uncovered certain proven facts, or, in some cases, unproven facts, which have shown us exactly just what makes these engines tick. Tick like the well-tuned grandfather clock that gives you the correct time minute after minute, day after day, week after week, month after month, and yes, year after year, even after you die and the ingrate of a nephew pawns it to pay off his gambling debt.

So what have we found out about these bodies? What is the key to our longevity? How do we do the amazing things we do? What makes it possible for our bodies to get up, and work every day, sometimes for little or no pay, or even less pay for the females of the species who also have bodies, but bodies that are admired not for their strength like male bodies are, but are admired like the male bodies aren't, in a creepy sort of way sometimes, not by me though, because I see bodies in a scientific way only having no sex, no color, no religion, and no meaning other than what goes in and what goes out. My concern, so to speak, is solely the ins and outs of our bodies. What, and how much do we need to go into our bodies to satisfy our animalistic needs, and then, what happens once these elements enter our bodies in an endless cycle of in and out, in and out, out and in, and vice versa? Any way you look at it, there is a lot of in and out going on concerning our bodies. So after numerous run on sentences, what is the mysterious thing, this noun, this elusive substance we need? Meditation? Deep massage? Sex? No, we don't need any of those things, or at least only need them once in a great married while. We can live meaningless lives without them. The one thing we must have and want..is....

NO MORE DAMN ELECTORAL COLLEGE!! Yes, and FUEL! We need fuel.

Just like any other non-perpetual motion machine, we need fuel to run. But "why," the simple son might ask? We answer him by telling him that in this life, we are basically animals, and as animals, we need to keep healthy for all the things that animals do. In the case of Earth dwellers, (scientists have learned that the following is not necessarily true in other solar systems), we eat food, and drink liquids to keep us chugging along. We need a certain amount of calories a day to stay alive. We need calories (food) to go to work, to play, to open the doors that need opening, and the drawers that need drawing. We need calories to build the houses, run the companies, to keep the 1% the 1% and the other 99% hanging on by a thread. We need this fuel to do all we want to do, all we need to do, to be all we should be. But food alone, per se, is not enough.

What?!

That's right, we need white, red, green, brown, orange, yellow and purple food in our personal eco-systems every week. Why? Just because I say so? Yes, but in addition, tests conducted by the Food Nutrition Study Institute of Autonomy, in modern, bright lit laboratories, show that most people who get absolutely no calories or nutrition, score very low on their S.A.T. tests and rarely get their driver's licenses on the first try. Calorie starved people are usually in bad moods, and may be found in fetal positions, sobbing in the canned goods aisle at the Piggly Wiggly. So get those calories! But get the them Color Diet Way.

TWO: QUICK WEIGHT LOSS

In this crazy work-like-a-maniac madcap frenzy we call "life", we demand that things happen quickly. Fast foods, electric toothbrushes, hamburger helper, drive-through funeral visitations, and mobile apps. Apps that direct you to more apps are an indication of the on-going trend of this post-haste, vroom-vroom society. The Color Diet App. (short for Appetite), could actually help you lose enough weight in a week to be almost dead.

THREE: GOOD TASTING FOOD

We all are on a diet, because a "diet" is what we eat. But now that word implies that we have to give up something and eat something else. But, who wants to replace food that we love, with food that we don't? If the food on your diet doesn't look good, smell good, or taste good going down, what's the point? You might as well be a reporter on your high school paper. That said, it's a fact that some of the diet foods you are told to eat don't even resemble what we think of as "food."

The Color Diet, on the other hand, allows a dieter to eat regular, natural, every day, genuine, spontaneous food. Food that was food when granola was just a snappy Mexican dance to welcome the harvest. Our food looks like food is supposed to look, how it was meant to look and smell. It tastes like the food grandma used to make when she was alive. There are no additives, harsh chemicals, sub-joiners, pesticides, MSG's, GMO's or PCB's.

And because you eat only one color a day, you never see a clashing of colors on your plate, which could sicken you with huexia* and make you all peelie-wallie.

Remember the old parable? God, on the seventh day, a Sunday, during a round of golf with Buddha, asked: "Bude, what you think of my creation?" Buddha sunk a three mile putt, looked down upon Earth, and made some wisecrack about all the clashing colors. God said: "Oh yeah?" Buddha calmly said it wasn't a criticism, it was just an observation. God said: "Well, observe *this!*" and gave him the finger. It's an old parable but I thought I should include it here, because I need at least another 25 pages.

*Huexia is a real term. Look it up.

FOUR: SIMPLICITY

One of the reasons the Color Diet works is that besides being the only diet that should be taken seriously, it is *simple* *.

One of the first things a child learns is color. You can readily see this by the kind of food they throw on the floor. It's usually a color that doesn't fit in with the scheme. So it stands to reason that color is a theme in our lives from early childhood on. Perhaps, even before childbirth when the mother is supplying nutrition to her fetal scion.

In the Color Diet, there are seven basic colors. This is because there are seven different enzymes in your stomach, each having a color corresponding to the color of foods we recommend. These enzyme receptors are found not only in the stomach, but also on the tongue, glottis, epiglottis, supraglotis, and the glottis submajore.

In case you were unaware, color is described as the result of reflecting light. So how do we know what color the enzymes are? When they are in the fresh air, we see the colors. We've all heard the "if a tree falls in the forest, and no one is there, is there sound?" Bodily enzymes are like that, except the question would be: If a color is in the dark, is there still color? And the answer is: "Yes, you idiot!" Sorry, I'm not talking about you. You aren't an idiot, all the other people reading this are.

So, yeah, color. It's a colorist's job to make up colors, or, as they like to think, *discover* new colors. "Granny Smith green", "inchworm mauve", "cotton candy pink", and "denim blue" are just a few of the colors discovered just within the last 50 years. Colorists are like astronomers. There may be millions of new colors out there just as there may be millions of new planets out there also. Personally, I think we've run out of colors, but who knows? Scientists? No, not them. They have to find new medications for made up diseases so they can fulfill their commitment to big pharma. Buddha? Does he know? Probably, but he's not talkin'. Commodity traders? Maybe. But all the research isn't in yet.

Thankfully, the Color Diet sticks to seven basic colors. You'll never have to look for Crimean Red Peppers at the store, nor have to stock "Gobi desert brown sugar" in your house/cabin/or time share. There is a point, and anyone can see it, where brown ends and green begins. And it doesn't even matter if you are totally color blind, because what difference does it make if you think you are eating brown food, and you are actually eating orange, because as long as you eat only one color a day, you are a-ok.

- "Simple" As in Simple Simon met a pie man going to the fair". If I might, I've always wondered since I've heard this politically charged ditty, who was going to the fair, Simon, or the pie man? At any rate, if Simon was on our diet, the story may have gone like this:

SIMON: Pie man, mayest I have one of your finest Eskimo pies?

PIEMAN: But of course young simpleton.

SIMON: But coulds't you, kind purveyor, find it in your joyless heart to remove the chocolate surrounding the vanilla goodness?

PIEMAN: No chocolate?! You beef-witted, flap mouthed knave! Art thou a racist? (remember, the story is a political poem)

SIMON: Nay nay good pie man, I canst eat of the chocolate, for I am partaking of the new Color Diet, and today I eat only white victuals!

PIEMAN: Oh ho! Why of course my simple knotty-pated boy. Wouldn't you joineth my fellow pie men in a killing of the king, and then the shagging of his daughter, the princess?

FIVE: SUPPORTIVE FAMILY AND FRIENDS

Who loves the dieter? Pretty much no one. Dieters make non-dieters feel guilty about food lust, and their ungodly gorging. That writ, let's speak to the most difficult part of this or any other diet.

With every diet, no matter how inane, the dieter needs support. No matter how committed your are, no matter how much you want to lose weight, no matter what your New Year's resolutions are, you can't do it all by yourself. Sure you can feel better about dieting, or be satisfied by the results of the diet by looking at yourself in one of those trick mirrors in department store changing rooms, or by treating yourself to a mud and horse sweat facial, but you know in the final analysis, you will need confirmation of your success from loved ones or twos. You need a mate to cheer you on, grandparents to watch you chew, that nanny to tell you how terrific you look while she suckles your infant (on the infant's white day).

If you don't have that help, you might end up eating with people who are not interested in supporting you and your diet. Why? Because most people, being human, with human parts, needs, hopes, wants, regrets, ambitions, thirsts, yens, foibles, hankerings, and yes, even insatiable carnal desires, really want you to stay fat because it makes them feel thin.

Just the other second, a friend, who shall remain anonymous, told me that when he was having dinner with his ex, she offered him another helping of her delicious mashed potatoes with port wine, and coulis patfwa gravy.

He thanked her but said he couldn't eat another bite. I told him: "good for you Bob Goldenport!" But then he told me that she laughed and said: "oh posh, it's not heathy to be too thin", and dumped another soup spoon-full of potatoes on his plate. Then she said, as she took another bite of radish: "Besides, I like a man with a little meat on him." My friend, who has a great sense of humor, told me he said: "yes, I agree, I also like a woman with a little meat on her too", then he took one of the short ribs she hadn't touched, and gently placed one on her head and said: "yep, you *do* look better with a little meat on you. Obviously, their relationship was over so I did the right thing and asked him for her phone number. (Just kidding Jennifer, your's is the only phone number I want or need. I would never call, much less eat alone with another woman. Unless you decided we should have an open marriage, WHICH I'M NOT SAYING WE SHOULD, but if *you* wanted one, and it would make *you* happy, then I would consider it.)

Unsupportive people, out of jealousy, may encourage you to not continue your diet. They might tell you that dieting is unhealthy, and you should be proud of your body, that you've been tricked by the media, and that stores now have very stylish circus tents in all sizes. It's your decision. You don't have to listen to the people who might tell you that the Color Diet is unfit for human, animal, or even plant consumption. They might even recommend phony, alarmist websites that claim that the Color Diet is a scam, a sham, a fraud, s total waste of your hard-earned cash, dangerous, and may even lead to death. Don't listen to them because what makes the Color Diet so swell in any company is you can mash potato pie ala mode your head off on your white day. You can eat pure lard on your yellow day, or an entire chocolate cake with chocolate frosting on your brown day. Now, if someone says: Let's go for ice cream,instead of saying: I'd love to but I'm on a diet, so I can't, you can say: Yahahooieeee! Nummies! I'll bring a bucket, so let me at it! You can have a carton of vanilla if it's your white day, or have two chocolate brown cows on your brown day, a pistachio delight on your green day, strawberry frappe on your red day, banana ice cream on your yellow day, and a grape shake on your purple day. You may have to settle for orange sherbet on your orange day, but even if someone hands you a tubful of crisp, deep fried chicken skins, and it's your brown day, by all means, go ahead! There is literally no other diet on Earth or any other planet where fried chicken skins are on the "eat this" list.

Naysayers

As long as people say things, there will be people who will say: "nay!" Warning: beware of these sayers of "nay" for they might try and dissuade you from buying this book, or even suggest you don't recommend it to others. Look out for these thoughts from alarmists.

1. "IGNORE AUTHORS WHO TELL YOU THAT THERE ARE QUICK FIXES."

    A "quick fix?" What in heaven's gate does that mean? To us, "quick" means "right away". For example: "Come here quick!" That expression means drop what you are doing and get there Now!. Or "Quick! Duck!", which means that either something is coming at your head, or that you should shoot your gun to kill the mallard that is flying by.

    The Color diet *is* a quick fix." It starts to work when you buy the book, take it to your home, half-way house, or your tent under the freeway, and open the book to the first page.

2. "DON'T LISTEN TO DIETS THAT USE A SINGLE PRODUCT OR REGIMEN"

    There is a single product the Color Diet uses. This product is called "food." We're not sure what the word "regimen' means. We think that they may have misspelled "regiment", which is a unit in the armed forces like the Big Red #1, or the Green Berets, both of which are colors in the Color Diet book, in which case someone can expect a lawsuit headed their way.

3. SOME HEALTH EXPERTS SAY: "DON'T BELIEVE CLAIMS THAT SOUND TOO GOOD TO BE TRUE, OR SIMPLISTIC CONCLUSIONS DRAWN FROM COMPLEX STUDIES."

    Hooey, rot, fake news, and horsepucky. As long as we're at it, add a backhoe load of balder. The Color Diet's claims are not too good to be true, they are too true to be too good. Wait. They are not too true to be good, they are too too truly good. Makes little sense but what does make any sense now a days. It's not complex. It's a simple diet, with a simple theory, for simple people like you and me.

4. A CERTAIN TV DOCTOR SAID IN ONE OF HIS PROMOTIONS FOR HIS PROFIT-MAKING ENDORSEMENTS: "JUST BECAUSE THERE ARE 'STUDIES' ON THE DIET, DOESN'T MEAN THAT THE STUDIES ARE MEANINGFUL. WHAT IS MEANINGFUL IS THE PRODUCTS I PROMOTE ON MY TV SHOW."

    I'm not going to give the name of the 'doctor" in question, but let me tell you this: Last night I turned on my kitchen faucet and out came **ooze**, followed by a **doz**en fro**z**en pieces of mat**oz**.

    I've done so many studies, most of them double blind, and some triple blind, testimonials proving the color diet theory as fact. I tried listing all these facts on the internet, but at some point, the sheer number of them shut down the internet for a day, prompting a call from the internet asking me to stop listing all the facts. So we stopped, which is why you won't be able to find all that information on your computer.

5. "UNLESS THE DIET HAS TV ADS, DON'T FALL FOR IT.'

We don't have to advertise. We rely on "word of mouth" because isn't that where the food goes? These "people" you see in ads, who say they have tried this or that diet are not actual people. They are actors who are playing people. The people who recommend, by word of mouth, our diet are so real, that they are unattractive, and have speech impediments. They are 110% grade A, USDP inspected people. Chances are, if a person is good looking, can talk without starting over ten times, pronounces both "r"'s in library, and is trying to sell you something, they will be an actor or actress who is getting paid to say whatever they are told to say, while in reality, they have never tried the product, never will try it, and have been trained in the art of lying, otherwise known as "acting.

6. "DON'T BELIEVE DIETS THAT IGNORE DIFFERENCES AMONG INDIVIDUALS, OR GROUPS"

Wait a gosh darn millisecond. "Differences among individuals or groups?" Even though it's harder now-a-days, with intermarriage, inter-sexual species, and/or makeup, we can still tell the difference between men and women, miniature schnauzers, turtles, or lawyers and people.

The salient point here is that…basically, there is no difference. We are all human. "Difference" is what keeps us from uniting as one. Golfers or Democrats, aliens or Earthlings, we are all the same. Except for the aliens, they are from another planet, but, actually, if you extend oneness to the universe, then they just might be the same.

7. MAKE SURE YOU CHECK OUT CLAIMS OF FAD DIETS BY GOING TO A WEBSITE THAT CHECKS OUT FAD DIET CLAIMS."

We don't recommend that, but sure, go ahead, if you are that kind of nit-picking, information-highway slave. The Color Diet theory has not be futed, or re-futed by any scientific organization, or scientific person. In fact, many scientists we know, have been on the Color Diet and have incorporated it into their otherwise stunted lifestyle. If you think the Color Diet is a "fad" diet, you are wrong. You are wronger than wrong. In fact, you are almost criminally wrong. You are living in a dream world, so much so, that when you "wake up" you are not really awake, but dreaming that you are awake, and when you actually do wake up, you still are not sure if you are asleep or awake. The Color Diet slaps you in the face and says: "WAKE UP!

It's true. Seriously. May God give me the heebily-jeebilies before the next page if it's not.

Well, here we are at the next page, and I feel fine.

The Seven Basic Colors

We all know there are three basic colors, Red Green and something else. But according to Brit Nitsky, who used to name crayon colors for some of the biggest crayon companies in the world, says that there are some 30,000 variation and permutations of those three colors. 30,000!. And he goes on to say that, like snowflakes, no too colors are alike. "Even that brown crayon you may have used on your "my Little Pony" coloring book changes micron-scopically each time you put it down and then pick it up and use it again. The air, humidity, temperature, and even the air pressure have minute effects on the color. Britsky goes on to say that you can only see the subtle changes on his mitro-chronoscope which he says he has invented. He goes on to say: "No one should try and duplicate my machine, because if they did try, it would blow up in their faces. I have the plans, and they are carefully guarded by my poison science gnomes at my secret location in a cave near nowhere. THEY ARE NOT IN MY MOM'S BASEMENT, SO DON'T EVEN BOTHER LOOKING!. The plans are written in a complex invisible code. If you think for a second that you might be able to torture me and get the codes, I will only say that better and more efficient torturers than you have tried, and failed. Yes, I've been laughed out of many color conventions, and even though I am temporarily in a special restraining jacket, I will never quit my crusade! NEVER! Even if my theory is again rejected by the World Color Conference of Tinters, I will, and I swear this on a stack of dissertations, I will eventually disrupt the time/color continuum, and rule the world! HAHAHAHAHAHA!!

Wow. But for our Color Diet's sake, there are exactly seven basic color groups of food. Other than these seven, there are no other combinations that should ever enter your body. LET'S GO TO THE COLORS!!

WHITE AND TRANSPARENT

WHITE COLORS

Pearl, Ghost, Smoky, Baby Powder White, Ivory, Alabaster, Egg Shell White, Bone China White, Pale White, Vanilla, Cream, Seashell White, Slappy White, Betty White, Antique White, Scandinavian White, Snow White, Whitehead White, Whitehouse White, White Elephant White, White Collar White, White Hot White, Sheet White, Crest White, Whitecap White, Innocent White, Table Cloth White, Aspirin White, White Out White.

WHITE BENEFITS:

The Enzyme found in white foods is good for brain tissue. Morons, idiots, and racists, simply do not eat enough white foods. In this group you can find chicken, some fruits, some vegetables, breads, rice, some cheeses, dairy, and sugars. Some unenlightened people might say that in the long list of white foods, we have some of the blandest foods a person can put in their digestive system, which is the beauty of this genre of foods. Your white day will also give your digestive system a day off. Take a look at the list, you'll see foods that are pretty much digested as soon as they hit the lips. Some begin breaking down on the spoon or fork seconds before putting them in your mouth. That's how digestible this food group is. .

WHITE FOODS

Sugar,
Salt
Farina
Cottage Cheese
Egg Whites
Mushrooms
Raw Potatoes
Mayonnaise
Vodka
Gin
Perrier
Breads w/o Crust
Hearts of Palm
Alfredo Sauce
Salfredo Sauce (Alfredo's brother)
Vanilla Pudding
Parsley Root
Banana
Chicken Breast
White Wine That Looks More
White Than Yellow In A Glass
White Sodas
Most Skinned Apples
Marshmallows
Popped Corn
Cauliflower
Vanilla Pudding
Cream Cheese
Cottage Cheese
Parmesan Cheese
Provolone

Mozarella
Cool Whip
Kool Wip
Halibut
Tilapia
Cod
Haddock
Feta Cheese
Nom de la Feureau Cheese
Aspirin
Calcium Vitamins
Vitamin D-3
Banana
Onions
Oysters
Rice
Plain Yogurt
Garlic
White Pepper
Sour Cream
Oreo Cream Filling
Tofu,
Crisco
Mashed Potatoes
Turkey Breast
Wonder Bread (no crust)
Puffed Rice
Marshmallows
White Pepper
Elmer's Glue

RED

RED COLORS:

Cardinal, Salmon, Pink, Mauve, Crimson, Baboon Ass Red, Embarrassed Red, Fire Engine Red, Face Slap Red, In The Pink, Pink Belly Pink, Pig Pink, Primrose, Beet Rash Red, Rosacea Red, Scarlet Letter Red, Mars Red, Red Cent Red, Flame Red, Stop Light Red, Police Light Red, U. Of Wisconsin Red, Red Coat Red, Blood Red, Red Cross Red, Commie Red, Rouge Red, Red Grange Red, Ruby Red, Furious Red, Red Sky In Morning, Dark Sky at Night Red, Beet Red

RED BENEFITS:

Basically, Red Foods are needed for bigger lip width, and healthier looking genitals. After two weeks on The Color Diet, you should find your genitals looking like they did when you were a teenager, not haggard and gross like they do now. In fact, I would recommend taking a before and after picture. You and your friends will be amazed at the improvement.

The Red Group includes raw meats, vegetables, salmon, some sauces, Paprikas. and pink bubble gum.

RED FOODS

Tomatoes	Casillero
Red Pepper	Del Diaolo
Raspberries	Red Twizzlers
Strawberries	All Raw Beef
Ketchup	Cabernet Sauvignon 1914—2017
Apple Skins	Chili
Sangria	Kidney Beans
Pinot Noir	Most Barbecue Sauces
Raw Tuna	Pimentos
Salsa w/o Green Stuff In It	Tomato Soup

Cranberries
Tomato Bisque
Stewed Tomatoes
Sobor Tomatoes
V-8
Strawberry Splash Gushers
Cayenne Pepper
Raw Beef
Hot Dogs
Red/Rose Wine
Borscht
Red Beans
Beets
Red Trix

Red JuJubees
Pink Grapefruit
Ham
Globe Grapes
Salmon
Cherries
Raw Live
Pimentos
Cranberries
Corned Beef
Pomegranate
Paprika
Pink Grapefruit

GREEN

GREEN COLORS:

Artichoke Green, Asparagus Green, Dark Green, Fern Green, Forest Green, Jungle Green, Mint Green, Moss Green, Al Green, Green Tea, Teal, Olive Green, Green Recruit Green. Green Room Green, Greenland Green, Green Mountain Boys Green, Green House Green, Algae Green, Green Horn Green, Brian Green, Verdant Green, Shamrock Green, Sea Green, Pea Green, Aquamarine, Turquoise, Lime Green, Chantuse, Sea Sick Green, and Graham Greene Green.

GREEN BENEFITS:

Green food promotes healthier livers, and makes your hair easier to comb after a shower. Green means "GO!" and in this group, that's what you will do, because we are talking roughage. If you want to stay regular, and who doesn't, except extreme hoarders, I recommend the green group of foods. If you still are having problems priming the pump, so to speak, skip the yellow day and have a second green day. Green Day is a great band, and a green food is maybe the most important food group.

The Green Group includes most vegetables, unripe fruit, and moldy bread.

GREEN FOODS

Green Peppers
Kale
Lettuce
Celery
Pickles
Peas
Mint
Zucchini Skin
Spinach
Asparagus
Green Olives
Green Beans
Moldy Bread
Cucumber
Green Goddess Dressing
Avocado
Seaweed
Chives
Limes
Green Grapes
Moss
Mung Beans
Broccoli
Green Jello

Guacomole
Green Gummies
Lime Life Savers
Dillweed
Original Gatorade
Olives w/o Pimentos
Jalapeños
Oregano
Marjoram
Basil
Celery
Leeks
Bokchoi Leaves.
Honeydew Melon
Parsley
Thyme
Creme de Menthe
Okra
Brussels Sprouts
Spinach
Swiss chard
Fava Beans
Arugula

BROWN

BROWN COLORS

Tan, Hazel, Beige, Fawn, Chocolate Brown, Burnt Umber, Buff, Raw Umber, Russet, Sandy, Desert, Taupe, Mahogany, Sepia Burnt Sienna, Nut Brown, Brown as a Berry Brown, Poop Brown, Ground Brown, Fake Tan Brown, Lion Mane Brown, Chestnut Brown, Brown Out Brown, Smog Brown, Sandstorm Brown, and LeRoy Brown Is Back In Town Brown.

BROWN BENEFITS:

The Brown Enzyme helps build muscle, and will promote a healthy tan, longer eyelashes, and a good sense of humor.

This powerful group has the most fun foods in it, although every color group has its share. Chocolate, cocoa, coke, beer, and syrups make their debuts in this group. Coffee, and tea are the powerhouses of the Brown Group. Make sure you use brown sugar for either tea or coffee, and you'll have to take a pass on the cream, unless it's some chemically altered brown GMO laden Nestles™ concoction. I don't want to imply that Nesltes is evil. Not yet. I'm waiting for the big drought, when they corner the water market, and charge $17.50 for a bottle of tap water.

BROWN FOODS

Molasses	Kit Kat Bar
French Fries	Well Done Bacon
Pumpernickel (including the	Worstcesterhire Sauce
crust)	Spiced Rum
Potato Skins	Root Beer
Chocolate Milk	Cumin
Brown Rice	Bread Crusts
Cloves	Brown Jimmies
Death By Chocolate Cake	Sunflower Seeds
Turkey Leg	Peanuts

Flax Seed
Nutella
Fudge
Some Barbecue Sauces
Cocoa Puffs
Brown Mustard
Coffee (If Brewed with Brown Filters only)
Nutmeg
Lentils
Graham Crackers
Garbanzo Beans
Ginger
Coriander
Sage Jicama

Maple Syrup
Fudge
Whiskey
Dates
Figs
Some Raisins
Corn Flakes
Well-Cooked Meat
Soy Sauce
Peanut Butter
Gravy
Some Caviar
Cloves
Beer nuts

YELLOW

YELLOW COLORS:

Golden, Straw, Blond, Dyed Blond Yellow, Flaxen Yellow, Coward Yellow, Saffron Yellow, Sunny Yellow, Yellow Sea Yellow, Unhealthy Urine Yellow, Yellow Tail Yellow, Yellowstone Yellow, Yellow Jacket Yellow, Daisy Yellow, Yolk Yellow, Yellow Fever Yellow, Ol' Yeller' Yellow, Submarine Yellow, Mellow Yellow, "Yellow Everyone, How Ya All Doin? Yellow"

YELLOW BENEFITS

Yellow foods are responsible for building healthy bodies 12 ways, WWII, and a high tolerance for pain. Warning: It may confuse the "fight or flight" reflex. Cheeses, soups, squash, sweets and sours, many fruits, some vegetables, some dairy, and, of course, the star of this group, the egg yolk. Yellow is associated with the sun, and so it makes sense, that the yellow foods give a person the ability to tan quickly. They are usually full of Vitamin D, which is what the Sun is made of. Mostly. Really hot Vitamin D.

YELLOW FOODS:

Egg yokes
Yellow Cheese Fondue
Yellow Squash
Yellow Mustard
Corn
Yellow Honey
Butter
Lemonade
Yellow Grapefruit
Lemons
Cheap Champagne
Raw Pasta
Gold Fish Crackers
Yellow Onions
Yellow Mellow
Olive Oil
Canola Oil
Peanut Oil
Corn Oil

Applesauce
Challah
Margarine
Peaches
Pineapple
Yellow Dye #1
Yellow Peas
Mountain Dew
Chicken Soup
Mangos
Banana Pudding
    White Wine That Looks Yellow
In A Glass
Buttermilk
Golden Raisins
Cheddar Cheese
Yellow Mustard
Matzo balls
Schmaltz

ORANGE

ORANGE COLORS

Tangerine, Orange, Pumpkin, Setting Sun Orange, Carrot Orange, Apricot Orange, Peach Orange, Some Tomatoes Orange, Persimmon Orange, Round as an Orange. Popsicle Orange, Pongee, Orange You Glad I Didn't Say Yellow, Orange.

ORANGE BENEFITS:

At first glance, the Orange Group looks like a weak sister on this diet, but a closer look, reveals that she is a W.O.M.A.N. Orange is good for the eyes, ears, nose, throat, and for living past your due date. Sweet potatoes, and yams are the most powerful and feminine food on any menu, any table, on any planet.

ORANGE FOODS

Apple Juice
Apricots
Cantaloupe
Caramel Corn
Orange Juice
Ginseng
Squash
Orange Crush
Cheetos
Marmelade
Tumeric
Orange Peppers
Orange Life Savers
Corn Tortilla Chips
Orange Ade

Orange Pekoe Tea
Sweet Potato
Yam
Pumpkin
Ranch Dressing
Tangerines
Tangellos
Navel Oranges
No Belly Button Oranges,
Peaches
Papaya
Dreamsicle
Babkayum
Cheese Whiz
Circus peanuts

PURPLE

PURPLE COLORS:

Thistle, Mulberry Purple, Mardi Gras Purple, Byzantium, Psychedelic Purple, Orchid Purple, Mauve, Purple Rain Purple, Deep Purple Purple, Purple Haze Purple, Grape, Purple Heart Purple, Royal Purple, Lilac, Snow Cone Purple, Blood Pudding Purple, Egg Plant Purple, Slurple Purple

PURPLE BENEFITS:

"Purple". If you say it 100 times in a row, you'll forget your name, address, and phone number. But what a powerful food group! The purple pigment, or rather enzyme, is wholly responsible for balance. Not only that, it keeps your eyeballs round. Best of all, purple foods give you the kind of handshake that might just get you that job you want. Purple is associated with royalty, that is why purple food is called the King of Foods. Purple foods give you confidence. The confidence to rule a city, a county, a country, or even the World!

PURPLE FOODS

Blood pudding	Grape Juice
Purple Asparagus	Blackberry Brandy
Purple Cabbage	Raisins
Purple Carrots	Purple Olives
Purple Figs	Purple Nipple Purple
Purple Grapes	Purple Tipped Belgian Endive
Purple Bell Peppers	Purple Currents
Purple Plums	Lavender
Eggplant	"Blue" Berries
Prunes	Grape Soda,
"Blue" Tortilla Chips	Grape Sno-Cones

NO-NO'S: SOME FOODS TO NEVER EAT ON THIS DIET.

There is a long list of foods you should never eat when on the Color Diet™. Here are some of them.

Apple Jacks	Coffeemate. (Just because the
Beef-a-Roni	ingredients will kill anything
Black Licorice (Nobody likes it	sentient)
anyway)	Chicken Catchatorre (I just real-
Cannolies	ized that Joe *Torre* was a *catcher!*)

Choriso
Chop Suey
Colby Jack Cheese
Ding Dongs
Dolly Madison Cream Filled
Twinkles
Doritos
Whole Eggs
Egg Rolls
Fish Sticks
Flavored Yogurt
Fried Rice
Gefilte Fish
Ice Cream Sandwiches
Kishkas

Vegetable soup
Omelettes
Oreos
Ravioli
Rice-a-Roni
Perogis
Pizza
Pop Tarts
Sausage
Snickers
Subway Sandwiches
Sushi
Tacos
Twinkies

Recipes

WHITE

TWICE BAKED DAIRY DISAPPOINTMENT

INGREDIENTS/UTENSILS

4 pieces of Swiss™ cheese
1 large tub of Summer cottage cheese
4 serving spoons Sweet and Sour Cream
1 glob cream cheese
2 shot glasses of heavy whipping cream (3 shots if the whipping cream is not heavy enough)
1 bag of pre-crushed large marshmallows
1 off-white chocolate rectangle
A snizzle of Kosher salt
A fistful of graduated sugar
3 white orchids (remove the stems)
Slide rule
The New York Times Book Review Magazine

INSTRUCTIONS:

1. Preheat an oven to around 300 to 500 degrees, depending what month it is and the state in which you live. (There is a danger of the recipe exploding, a "dairy nova", with an oven interior of over 300 degrees in the Florida Keys.)
2. In a large mixing bowl, startle the Summer cottage cheese.
3. As you add the sweet and sour creme, increase startling, to about 127 RPM's.
4. Introduce the salt and sugar.
5. Once they have gotten to know each other, set the bowl outside in the sun. If it's cloudy out, a tanning bed will do.
6. Take the Swiss cheese and wave it in the air for stiffening.
7. Dip the stiffened Swiss cheese in various parts of a brandy snifter filled with the heavy whipping cream, until the cheese is well snurdled.
8. Bury the cheese into the heavy whipping cream. This time for good.
9. Place everything into an oven-comfortable baking dish. With the slide rule determine the middle of the oven, and place the baking dish near it.
10. Cook from six to 20 minutes.
11. When the baking dish can be touched with your finger without raising a blister, remove, and set on a tile floor.
12. Read one New York Times book review.
13. Lay the off-white chocolate rectangle, and large pre-crushed marshmallows over the top of the warm commotion. The white chocolate should be in the middle and the marshmallows at right angles to the sides of the baking dish. (Note: If you can't find pre-crushed marshmallows in your area, regular marshmallows can be crushed by keeping them under an often-used sofa cushion for about a week)

14. Let cool to room temperature. Be sure it's a room temperature that the woman of the house likes, not the frigid one the man usually likes. The room for cooling should be a quiet dark room, perhaps the bedroom, under the bed, if it fits.
15. Serve in the baking dish at about 8 PM

YIELD: 8 large squares, 16 small squares, 32 bite sized squares, 64 miniature shapes, or, four teenager sized squares.

The disappointment? There aren't any leftovers.

COTTAGE FLOWER CHICKEN SMOOTHIE

INGREDIENTS/UTENSILS

2 bushes cauliflower
1/2 tub curd-free cottage cheese
1 large masonic jar chicken
preserves
7 thimbles of talcum powder.
A standard sewing thimble.

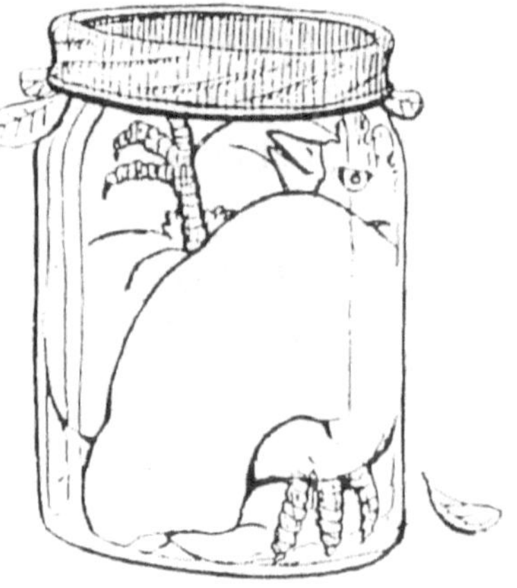

INSTRUCTIONS

1. Rotate the chicken preserves clockwise.
2. Remove the chicken from the jar.
3. Dry with a blow dryer.
4. Puree the cauliflower in a white plastic bowl.
5. Mix the cottage cheese and cauliflower until you can't tell which is which.
6. Bone the chicken.
7. Don't tell anyone.
8. Set the stovetop burner to really hot.
9. Dump the mixture into a saucy pan.
10. Put the pan with the mixture in it on the really hot burner.
11. Heat for what seems to be a long time. Say, for instance, like you are in a doctor's office, waiting for a prostate exam.
12. Don't take your eyes off the pan because you want to remove it just before the bubbles pop.
13. Then remove from the stove, and let sit over-night.
14. In the morning, before noon, scoop the chicken, cottage cheese, and cauliflower into a blender. Set on mulch.

15. Mix in the talcum powder, and drink plain, or pour over
    pieces of white bread.

(Talcum has some beneficial minerals like magnesium silicate!)

YIELD: The EPA recommends less than one, but who's to know?

POKY CHICKEN GUMBO

INGREDIENTS/UTENSILS

The white meat from a small chicken
2 dozen egg Whites
1 white wine
1 whitefish, the whiter the better.
White out.
A large white bowl

INSTRUCTIONS:

1. Mix all ingredients separately.
2. Put the mixture in the bowl.
3. The mixture should be only 3/4's the way up the bowl to allow for expansion.
4. Put the mixture in the refrigerator.
5. In 15 minutes take the mixture out of the refrigerator.
6. Wait 5 minutes and put the mixture in again.
7. Then you take the mixture out.
8. You put the mixture in and you shake it all about
9. You make the chicken gumbo
10. And you stir it all around,
11. That's what it's all about!
12. You make the chiiiicken gumBO
13. You make the chiiicken gumBO
14. You make the chiiicken gumBo
15. That's what it's all about.
16. Garnish with tofu.

YIELD: Way too much.

CONNESTOGA PORK CHIFFLAUT

Before we delve into this recipe, we need to talk a little about probably the most intelligent animal in filmdom, the Pork, which, of course includes that endearing, yet politically incorrect character in Disney cartoons, none other than the stuttering, Mr. Porky the Pig.

Once thought of as a filthy animal fit as food for neither Jew nor Muslim, it is now considered a clean, adorable household pet. I myself can't look at this purveyor of loins, chops, and bacon, without thinking that in the animal world, this "pig" as some would have it, should only come out in public if it is resting comfortably on a spit over a pit of flaming charcoal. Roast it, bake it, pull it, anyway you do it, the pig is meant to be eaten.

But it is true that pork is a food that must be cooked properly to avoid digestion problems such as trichinosis, long worms, hook worms, book worms, abominable phlegm, bleet, and/or gaucherie.

But with today's careful slaughter (more like a holocaust) of the oinker, we don't have to worry about how we cook what we call: "swine."*

The Connestoga Pork recipe is completely safe. It is rated PG (pretty good) as far as the USDA ratings go, although it isn't recommended for children under 1 or adults over 100.

This treasured recipe has been handed down through the ages and is an integral part of the Color Diet.

Here's the story: Settlers would sometimes have to eat their pigs when other food wasn't available on their long trek westward. And, as we know, they were loath to build fires, because the smoke from a fire might alert their enemies, the drunken, sex starved U.S. Calvary soldiers.

So what to do? Starve? No. They, instead of starving to death, which would have hindered their progress West, they invented a method of cooking pork without having to build a fire.

Here's how: Sometimes on the prairie, temperatures would rise above 100 degrees. I think the saying went: "Hot enough to fry an egg on the back of a hairless dog".

One pioneer, John something, got the idea to wrap a small pig in a heavy blanket and put it on top of a wagon so the sun would do what sun's do best. Slowly heat things to "hot as hell". You may not know this, because I certainly didn't until I made it up, that pigs can withstand temperatures as high as 180°, which is about what it reaches when you are wrapped in a blanket in 100° heat on top of a Connestoga Wagon. So, the swine is pretty comfortable while the heat kills the microbe-protho organisms, and worms, that can only stand temperatures of under 150°.

The heat also mendles the flesh of the pig, making it totally fit to eat.

At night, while the pig wasn't looking, they would kill it with an overdose of tranquilizers, eat the mendled pig, get high on the tranquilizers still in the pig, then settle down for a good night's sleep under the warm blanket used to cook the pig.

*"Swine" Definition from Webster: Any of various stout-bodied short-legged omnivorous artiodactyl mammals with a thick bristly skin and a long flexible snout; Then: "a contemptible human". Obviously, an insult to the pig.

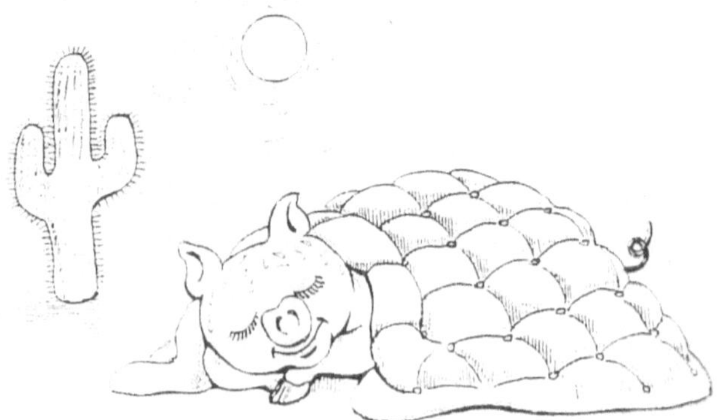

INGREDIENTS:

1 45 pound piglet. (Always use the piglet, a full-grown pig is
sub-digestible.)
A bag of red peppers
Large turkey baster.
Cayenne pepper
2 Red licorice sticks.
1 Tablespoon liquid Sominex
Food scraps (anything)
1 small pig trough
I can of Pillsbury Kentucky Corn Mash.™

INSTRUCTIONS:

1. Set the oven to 180°. Remove all the broiler pans, trays, and
   racks.
2. Mix the Sominex™ in a small bowl.
3. Add corn mash.
4. Use the turkey baster to feed to the piglet.
5. When Piglet gets drowsy, place in pig trough.
6. Set the trough with the Piglet on the bottom of the oven. (A 15
   to 20 pound piglet should fit comfortably into most standard
   ovens).
7. Turn off the oven light, it's hard to look at a piglet who's won-
   dering what's going on.
8. Put all the other ingredients in a bowl. Cover with Saran Wrap™
   Or a tarp.
9. Leave the house while the piglet is chifflauting just in case it
   wakes up.
10. Leave the piglet in the oven for *at least* 8 hours. When you
    come home, the piglet should be fully awake, dark pink to red,
    and famished.

11. In the trough, put the red peppers, cayenne pepper, licorice sticks and an overdose of any barbiturates, if you have something on hand, fine, otherwise any vet can sell you methyl-proloxade, which is used to put animals down whether they are ready or not.
12. The piglet will eat all the ingredients, including the juices in which it had been chafflauted, basting it from the inside out.
13. When the piglet has expired, put it back into the oven, and roast for two more hours at 450°.
14. Let the piglet "breathe" before slicing. When slicing, serve only the pink chafflauted flesh, which is the tenderest of the pork. If by some fluke, you over cook the piglet, and it is browned, put it in the refrigerator and serve on your Brown Day.
15. Season to taste.

Yield: 15 hongry buckeroos.

CHEWED WIENER TORTE MOLD

INGREDIENTS/UTENSILS

1 cup chewed wieners

2 lbs. Rhubarb

3 cups rounded pot of borscht

4 Tbsp. Of Schmucker's cherry jam (not the jelly)

5 Tbs. Paprika

6 capon chicken heart

7 small beets

8 pimentos

9 Globe Grapes (including seeds)

10 Downing Street.

INSTRUCTIONS:

1. Set the oven at right angles to the refrigerator. Turn oven to 650°
2. Saute rhubarb in the cherry jam, and turn the oven down to 500°
3. Sprinkle the chewed wieners gradually over the rhubarb mix.
4. Grease a small card table until slippery enough to slide a quarter from one end to the other.
5. Spread the wiener mix thinly over the table.
6. Put the paprika away.
7. Drink the Borscht
8. Mash the rest of the ingredients in a bowl from Sur le Table™
9. Throw a paper tablecloth over the wiener mix. Let sit for two episodes of Seinfeld.

We have some time now, we'll let the mold settle, and be right back after this:

(PAID ADVERTISEMENT)

ANNOUNCER: Sur Le Table, your one stop shop. Everything for a person who wants to be able to tell people that you shopped at a place with a French name, and that maybe you can speak French.

(GENERIC KITCHEN)

(TWO WOMAN DRINKING STRAIGHT OUT OF BOTTLES OF GIN)

IST WOMAN: Gwen, that pie is perfect!

2nd WOMAN: It's because I got the pie pan from Sur la tawb lah.

1st WOMAN: Oooooh, I wish I could shop there, but I don't speak French.

2nd WOMAN: Hahahaha…

ANNOUNCER: You'll get the best in cookware, no matter what language you can't speak.

SLIDE: THIS WEEK, SALE ON ALL "QUALET DU MARCHEAT" EGG BASTERS!

Hey, we're back and our mix is now ready for the next step for your Chewed Wiener Torte Mold.

10. Take the table by both sides, and turn it upside down.
11. Roll up the cloth
12. Freeze
13. Serve cold on red acoustic tile.
14. Turn off the oven.

Yield: One family of from 3 to 9.

MINI STRONI AL FONGOOL

INGREDIENTS/UTENSILS

¾ Roma Tomato skinned.
½ Red Pepper
½ cup Campbell's Tomato Soup
Smimch of Red Dye #2 or #3.
1 Red Savino Habanero Pepper
1 Trinidad Moruga Scorpion Pepper
1 Komodo Dragon Pepper.
1 Ghost Pepper

2 Drops Pure Capsaicin.
Paprika
You will also need:
A pair of plastic fire retardant gloves
HazMat Suit™
Goggles
24" Fan
Titanium bowl.
Ice Bag.
Hammer
Small Fire Extinguisher
First Aid Kit
Heavy duty lawn/garbage bag.
Two Concrete Blocks.

INSTRUCTIONS:

1. Clear the house of any living thing, including plants.
2. Empty the refrigerator.
3. Open all windows and doors.

4. Turn the fan on, and face it in the direction of the work space.
5. In the Rubber Ice Bag insert the red pepper, tomato soup, red dye #2 or #3, and Roma tomato.
6. Using the rolling pin, squash the ingredients in the bag.
7. Squeeze the ingredients from the bag into the titanium mixing bowl. *
8. Don the HazMat™ suit
9. Then, making sure your gloves are securely tied to the suit, place the rest of the ingredients into the bag.
10. With five or six deft blows, hammer the ingredients in the ice bag into submission.
11. Pick up the bag, place it over the mixing bowl, resting the bag on the rim of the bowl.
12. Wait two minutes until the mixture has melted a hole into the ice bag and deposited its ingredients into the bowl. Don't worry about getting rubber from the bag into the bowl, the peppers will have vaporized the rubber which is what causes the mixture to fall into the bowl.
13. Carefully cover the bowl with a metal lid.
14. Open the refrigerator door.
15. Very slowly and carefully, pick up the bowl, *** and place it in the refrigerator.
16. Wait 24 hours to let the mixture settle in the refrigerator.
17. Serve cold directly from the metal bowl. Do not try and serve on a plate or any other utensil other than the bowl.
18. Tell your guest, that it's best to tip the bowl and drink it directly from the bowl.
19. Video tape your guest's reaction. Try and catch the bulging eyes, which is always hysterical.
18. After dinner, take the plastic bag and insert your guest's body with the concrete blocks into it.
19. Put it in trunk.

20. Drive to the harbor.

21. Dump mixture into the harbor.

Yield: Enough to serve one person who has insulted you or your family in any way. Ever..

*Don't use plastic utensils for this recipe

***If mixture is moved too quickly or jarred in any way before it goes into the fridge, it might explode.

GREEN

EASY PEEZY, HOT AND SQUEEZY
CRUMBLED AVOCADO SKINS

The healthiest part of the avocado? The pit? No! It's a deadly poison. The meat? Very healthy, but not quite as nutritious as the skin! Yes, the skin. My Mom, Beatrice Chudnow-Goldberg used to ask: "You aren't eating the crusts? That's the healthiest part! You're not eating the potato skin? It's the healthiest part of the potato!" And "I've scrambled the eggs with the shells, because the shells are the healthiest part of the egg and it will give you beautiful bowel movements."

It's the same with the avocado skins. There are more vitamins and nutrients in one avocado skin than in twelve Flintstones "Complete" Vitamins™.

The following recipe is just a healthier variation of the potato skins you can order at TGI Fridays, or Chili's or any of the other "we have microwaved food for everyone and anyone, especially if you can't afford nice restaurants" restaurants.

INGREDIENTS/UTENSILS

4 Average sized avocados. An "average" avocado should fit in the palm of a grown woman.
A Pinchette of dill weed
2 things of broccoli.
A leaf from the bokchoi plant
Green Jello
3/4 brandy snifter of pickle juice.

INSTRUCTIONS:

1. Heat the oven (broil) to 570°.
2. Using a #7 pastry brush, coat the insides of the halved avocado

skins with the pickle juice. (Don't worry about over-coating, because most of the juice will be absorbed by the skins, and the excess with be absorbed by the high heat of the oven)

3. To prevent creebling, pre-gest the broccoli, and egest it into a champagne flute
4. In a fireproof bowl, hobnob the ingredients.
5. When ingredients are totally acquainted, put bowl on the upper rack.
6. In about a half hour, using the fireproof gloves, turn the bowl 25 degrees (always turn a heated bowl clockwise).
7. Then every 1/2 hour, turn the bowl another 25 degrees.
8. In four hours, remove the bowl. Set it on a granite or cement counter top.
9. Let cool for two hours.
10. When cool eat directly out of the bowl. You can't refrigerate or save this recipe as leftovers.

Yield: It depends on how much your dinner audience weighs, but the final product should feed 4 children of medium height and weight, or 1 lumberjack.

STUFFED PECK OF PICKLED PEPPER MOCK FONDU.

INGREDIENTS/UTENSILS

A Peck of Pickled Peppers, Pared.
5 Medium Mung Beans
4 Rounded Shots of Creme DeMenthe.
1 Quart of Green Goddess Dressing
1/2 cup of green jimmies.

INSTRUCTIONS

1. Remove the peppers from the package or bag.
2. Set the package or bag aside.
3. Rinse the peppers under running lukewarm water.
4. Place the peppers in a large cooking utensil with a close-fitting cover.
5. Put the utensil on the biggest burner of your stove.
6. Turn it on to almost full blast.
7. Bring it to a boil or abscess.
8. Let it sit, boiling until bored.
9. Puree the asparagus. Oh, I forgot to tell you that you'll need 12 asparagus sticks.
10. Set the asparagus in the top shelf of the refrigerator.
11. Turn burner up fuller.
12. Take the pureed asparagus out of the refrigerator.
13. Beat, blend, and chill
14. Slice, dice and shimmy
15. Mix, fix, and fold.
16. Manny, Moe, and Jack.
17. Find the package you set aside earlier. The one the peppers came in. Or, more grammatically, in which the peppers came.

18. Fill the bag or whatever with air, and pop it with a loud bang
    over the asparagus.
19. Slice the asparagus with the grain.
20. Flute the mixture.
21. Arrange carefully in a fondue pot.
22. Sprinkle with green Jimmies.
23. Put everything in a warm closet until all the ingredients get
    good and green, maybe 3 or 14 days.
24. Top the whole thing with Green Goddess dressing, and you are
    ready to eat this bizarre treat! You might want to serve it with a
    side bowl of green salsa.

YIELD: Who cares?

PARTY SEAWEED DIP

***INGREDIENTS: (The ingredients in this recipe can also be
used in WACKAMOLE GUACMOLE)***

4 large fronds of Pacific Ocean Kelp (you can find Pacific Ocean
kelp in any Asian grocery store west the San Andreas Fault.)
One box of lime Jello.™

INSTRUCTIONS:

1. Alternately dry and rinse the kelp in the sun for four or five
    days.
    All salt must be rinsed off before processing the kelp since salt
    is in the white food group. Kelp is very brittle when completely
    dried and salt free, so make sure you lay green construction
    paper under the kelp when drying it.
2. Crinkle the kelp into small, teeny tiny little pieces.
3. Make the lime Jello™ using a quarter cup more water than is
    called for on the box. The jello should be the consistency of
    skin foam. You would get the same consistency by squeezing
    the Jello™ through your teeth a lot like you used to do when
    you were a kid, and liked to play with your food (see "Patty
    cake patty cake: Playing With Your Food")
4. In an industrial strength blender (rentable at U-Haul™) murdle
    the Jello™ and kelp.
    The result will be a delightful paste ready for dipping with cel-
    ery, pickles, or asparagus spears.
    The Petri dish? A very clever kind of serving tray which will
    delight and bemuse your dinner audience.

YIELD: Four hungry gremlins, or six infants.

BROWN

RALPH STEW

INGREDIENTS/UTENSILS

Big honkin' five gallon pot.
1 pint heavy black strap molasses
1 cup Kellogg's Corn Flakes
2 cups soy sauce.
1 gallon chocolate milk.
3 cups diced pumpernickel bread.
1 Tbsp. Nutmeg
1 Tbsp. Cloves.
1 Gallon of your best whiskey or bourbon.

INSTRUCTIONS.

1. Get really drunk on the whiskey and/or bourbon.
2. Once sufficiently drunk, throw all the ingredients into the five gallon pot.
3. Drink from the pot.

YIELD: No one knows for sure.

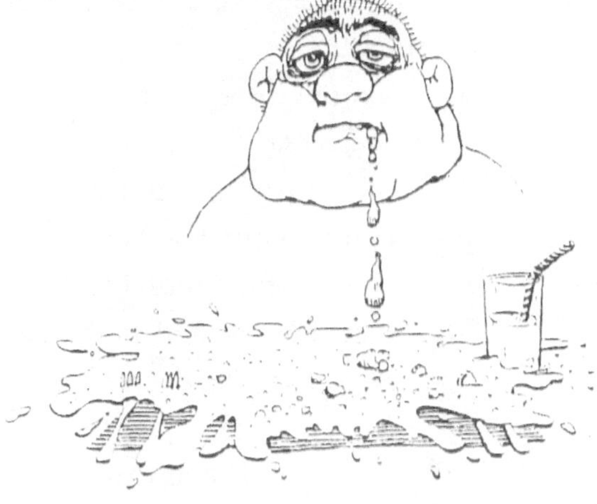

CHINESE CHOCOLATE LIVER BARS

INGREDIENTS:/UTENSILS

2 medium Hershey Bars™
1 bag ballpark salted outside the shell peanuts
1 lb. Calf's liver
2 cups soy sauce
Acetylene Torch
6 tongue depressors

INSTRUCTIONS:

1. Melt the Hershey bars over a low flame about an inch high., Be sure to use some sort of container.
2. Mince or chew the peanuts until they make a fine paste.
3. Carefully fold the peanut paste into the Hershey mix.
4. Cook the liver until it's brown (remember, raw liver is in the Red Group).
5. Fold in the liver.
6. Divide the mixture into a muffin tin and stick a tongue depressor into each cup.
7. Put in your refrigerator freezer or outside if it's Winter, freeze overnight.
8. The next day, using your acetylene torch, heat the soy sauce to 1,750 degrees.
9. Take the preparation out of the freezer or the outdoors, and immediately pour the hot soy sauce over the bottom of the mold to release the individual bars from the muffin tins.
10. Top with tiny cocktail umbrellas, and eat cold, right off the depressors. Save the depressors for when you feel sick later.

YIELD: Anyone and/or anyone who's willing to try it.

FRISKY BEANS

INGREDIENTS/UTENSILS

1 Pound Mexican Jumping Beans
1 Cupule of Brown Hot Sauce.

INSTRUCTIONS

1. Pour the Jumping Beans onto a plate.
2. Pour the hot sauce on the Jumping Beans
    The hot sauce will invigorate the jumping beans and cause them to frolic about. The more sauce you add, the higher they jump.

YIELD: Depends. A lot of the beans might end up on the floor.

Also, there are a couple of games you can play with this dish.(See "PLAYING WITH YOUR FOOD")

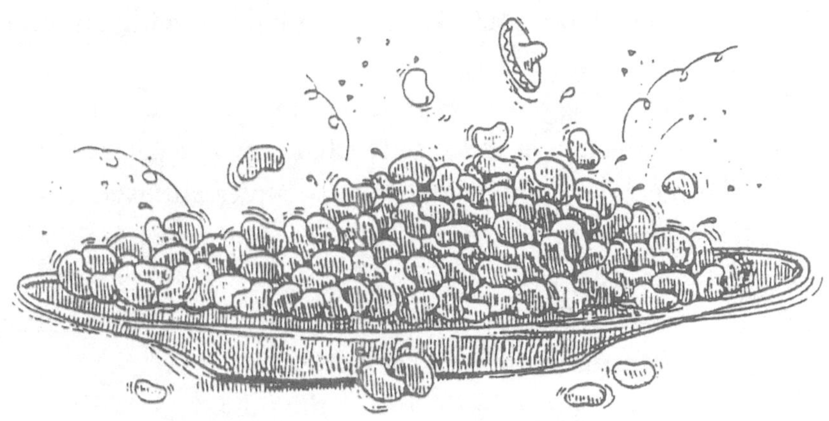

YELLOW

MOLTEN EGG PIE

INGREDIENTS/UTENSILS

750 Egg yolks
A dash of lemon juice.
Egg shells
Goggles
A bath tub
Tire inner tube
Aluminum siding
Rubber apron

INSTRUCTIONS

1. Wake up early.
2. Don't bother showering. Don't eat anything.
3. Dress in something you don't care about ever wearing again.
4. Lock the doors and cover the windows with aluminum siding.
5. Put on the goggles and rubber apron.
6. Prepare the lemon juice. Tell it that it will be combined with 750 egg yokes, and it might not be a pleasant experience.
7. Take a tube out of a car tire, or use a fresh tube from the Tub, Tube, and Beyond store.
8. In the bathtub, beat and berate the eggs. Call them names like "You stupid unborn cluckers!"
9. Siphon the eggs from the tub to the tube.
10. Put the tube into the car tire.
11. Drive around 20 miles at approximately 60 miles per hour,

or whatever is five miles above the highway speed limit. Try to not make any sharp turns, as this will stiffle the eggs.

12. If the outside temperature is above 79 degrees, the drive time will be shorter, as it will be if you are driving on asphalt as opposed to concrete.

13. Remove the tube from the tire. Squeeze the molten eggs into galvanized zinc pie plates.

14. Don't bother with a crust. The molten eggs would turn any crust into malgadust.

15. The pies must be eaten hot. Once cooled they are useless as food.

YIELD: 3 25 Lb. Pies.

INGREDIENTS/UTENSILS

Pot-o-honey.
A lot of mustard.
A huge chunk of your favorite cheese.

INSTRUCTIONS

1. With a wood plane, take a chunk of cheese, slice it paper thin.
2. Put some honey on it. Make sure you put the honey on first so the mustard doesn't fall off the cheese.
3. Put some mustard on the honey.
4. Stop when either you have enough, or your hands are covered with honey/mustard.

YIELD: How many Honey Mustard Thins are "enough"? You tell me.

As a bonus, if you have children who like to lick the spoon when you make cookies, let them lick your hands, they'll love it, and you!

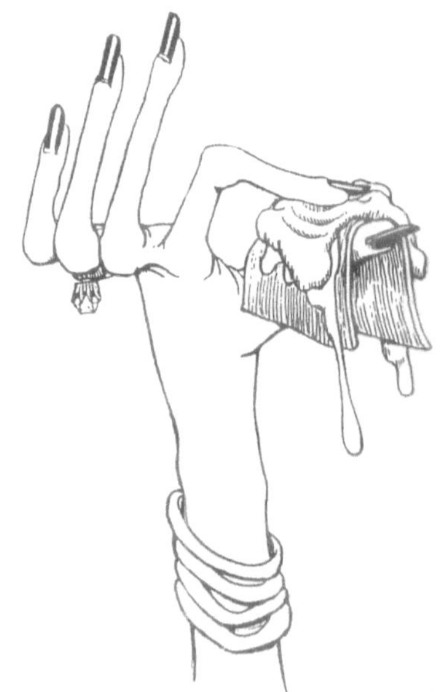

FROZEN HONEY MUSTARD THINS™.

INGREDIENTS/UTENSILS

Honey Mustard Thins™
A refrigerator with a freezer compartment, or a stand-alone freezer, or a patio in Greenland.

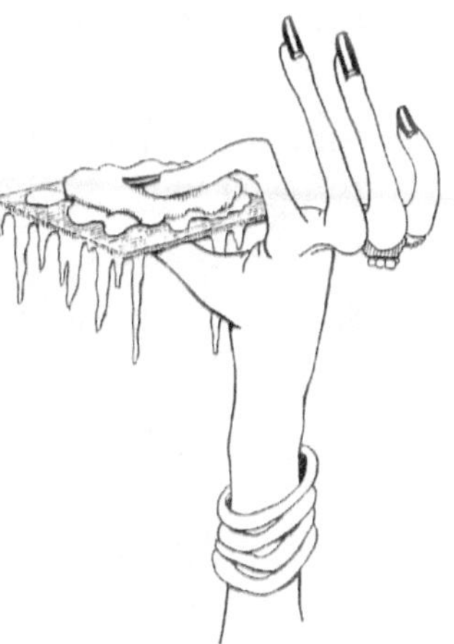

INSTRUCTIONS.

1. Put the Honey Mustard Thins™ in the freezer compartment of the refrigerator, stand-alone freezer, or the patio outside your house, or a neighbor's if you live in Greenland.
2. In 25 minutes, take out and eat like a Eskimo™ Pie or Popsicle.

COMFORTABLE BONANZA CHEESE HAT STRUDELETTES

INGREDIENTS/UTENSILS

A Green Bay Packer Cheese Head.
A 7 oz. Brick of any yellow cheese. We recommend Gouda.
American cheese is not goudanough.
1 cup of Hollandaise sauce.
Double boiler
Skinny crackers. Or straws. Or both.

INSTRUCTIONS:

1. From a tap, found in your kitchen (if you don't have a kitchen, use the garden hose) add a level quart of water into Double Boiler.
2. On an open flame, bring water to a roaring boil. Let it boil for at least five minutes
3. Put all the cheese in the top pan.
4. Let melt until the cheese looks cheesewhizish.
5. Make the Hollandaise sauce, or buy a bottle of it from your local grocer5. Very slowly add the Hollandaise dressing. It should take 10 or 15 minutes to add it.
6. Turn the heat down to between a low boil, and a simmer.
7. Line the holes in the cheesehead with foil. Any kind will do, aluminum or otherwise.
8. Remove the top boiler with the melted cheese.
9. Carefully pour the hot cheese into the cheesehead holes.
10. Let stand for some time.
11. Serve hot with skinny crackers.

YIELD: 7 fans if using the crackers, 3 if using the straws.

ORANGE

RUFFLED MANGO SOUP

INGREDIENTS/UTENSILS

A floor
Quart saucepan
4 ripe mangoes
1 quart water
An ice cube

INSTRUCTIONS:

1. Take an ice cube out of the freezer and set it aside.
2. Take the mangoes out of the fruit bin and listen to them. They should sound just right. If they do, then they are ready for Ruffled Mango Soup, or Knajga, as it is called. The national dish of the Crotes.
3. Start by dropping the mangos on the floor, or counter if you are over 7 feet tall.
4. Drop 12 to 13 times, just enough to ruffle them, not rile them. A height of 4 to 5 feet is recommended.
5. By this time the ice cube should be melted to perfection.
6. Scurdle the water in a saucepan, and heat to 95 degrees.
7. Very quickly slide the mangos into the hot, but not boiling water.
8. Let simmer for forty minutes to an hour, exactly.
9. You should have a very thick and delicious Knajga that can be eaten with a spork, or, serve it upright as a main course.
10. Use a towelette to dry the counter.

YIELD: Just enough.

SZECHUAN LOX

INGREDIENTS/UTENSILS

1 pound, Nova lox
1 pint sweet and sour juice.
1 cup cheese salsa
#1 tong
You will also need a 12X8 piece of well-rusted cast iron.

INSTRUCTIONS:

1. Take the one pound of Nova Lox, and using your #6 mangle, pound the lox even more. Pound them into thin, thin strips about 1/16 inch each.
2. Using a #1 tong, carefully dip each strip into the sweet and sour juice.
3. Lay each strip onto a piece of flat cast iron. (You can find flat cast iron at any scrap iron yard. If it isn't rusted, leave it in a large cask filled with water for about a week)
4. Completely soak a swatch of orange cloth (Use CookCo's™ Swatch Kit™ found at any Bed Bath and Beeeeeyoooooonddddd.™) with the sweet and sour juice.
5. Wring the cloth out over the lox.
6. Unceremoniously dump the entire jar of salsa over the lox.
8. Let sit.
9. And sit.
10. And sit, until the salsa completely dries up.

YIELD: 1/2 a Girl Scout™ troop™

CANTALOUPE RIND CORN CRISPS

INGREDIENTS/UTENSILS

1 small pumpkin

1 tablespoon of #3 orange zest. The zestier the better.

10 orange Chuckles™

30 medium Cheetos™

1/3 cup marmalade

You will also need a small flame thrower or torch.

A welder's mask

#3 stilleto

INSTRUCTIONS

1. With a #3 mangle, crush the Cheetos™
2. Then, with a rolling pin, roll the Cheetos™ into a fine powder, the consistency of un-sifted, bleached, partially refined flour.
3. Disorient the Cheetos™ with the marmalade.
4. Take the top of the pumpkin off. Cut around the middle of the pumpkin, but not exactly in the middle, maybe just where the pumpkin begins to curve inward.
5. Scoop the finely powdered Cheetos™ and dump them into the pumpkin.
6. With a #3 stiletto slice the Chuckles™ lengthwise into thirds.
7. Cover the mixture completely with the orange Chuckles™ The less Cheetos™ and marmalade you see the better.
8. Put on the welder's mask.
9. Take the torch, or the flame thrower (a torch you can buy at any hardware store would be fine), and light it.
10. Aim the torch or thrower in the center of the open pumpkin.
11. In the low mode, melt the Chuckles™ over the Cheetos™

Serve with stainless steel spoons. Stainless steel is grey, and therefore neutral, usable with any color food.

YIELD: One PTA meeting.

PURPLE

BLACK AND BLUE ETRUSCAN PIDDLIN'

Correct me if I'm wrong, but It's a pretty well-known fact that the ancient Etruscans had a highly advanced society. They were makers of fine terra-cotta, winsomely handsome sculpture, and Italian/Greek food. Their main contribution to the world is the invention of the Klamata olive. Just as the beautiful Etruscan art is displayed in museums around the world, the Klamata olive is proudly displayed on grocery shelves worldwide.

This recipe is dedicated to those fine people who reigned supreme from about 600 BC to just before Rome decided to kill anyone who wouldn't say: "I am Roman now", around 50 B.C.

INGREDIENTS/UTENSILS

Purple asparagus.

25 - 30 Raisins depending on the size.

(Do not use "Jumbo Raisins" because there will be all colors of raisins in the package, unless you want to pluck out the purple raisins.)

1 Large Aubergine Eggplant.

(The Aubergine Eggplant is the official eggplant of rich people, but if you don't tell them, you may use it also, as long as it's in a recipe, and you get rid of all the non-aubergine innards. You are allowed to display the plant on a shelf in your house to impress your guests).

Purple carrots.

One heaping German Beer Stein of blueberries.

One 16 oz. Jar of Kalamata olives

1 2 X 12 baking pan.

1 Oster Blender*

Oster™ is the world's finest blender. In mixing test after mixing test, people chose Oster over any other blender. I, myself,* *have the Oster Pro 1200 Blender 3-in-1 with attachment and XL Personalized Blending Cup™. "Oster™ - Legendary performance, Designed to last"

*Mention this mention at any store selling Oster products, and get 5% off on any Oster™ product!****

**I, personally, must be with you at time of purchase.*

INSTRUCTIONS:

1. Plug in your Oster Pro 1200™, to any electronical outlet. Admire those sharp, powerful true stainless-steel blades, those sleek, state of the art space age plastic contours.
2. With pride, put the olives into that fine Oster™ mixing machine.
3. Hobnob, then fuse the carrots.
4. Set on ™"Turbo". Put the handy heat-sealed rubber lid on, and set to puree. With a flick of a switch, you'll have olives that would be proud to be called puree.
5   Disorient the olives with the carrots.
6. Mingle the blueberries with the raisins.
7. Bardle them into the blender.
8. Keep the cover of the blender off, so the blueberries and raisins get a healthy infusion of air.
9. Pour all the ingredients into an ungreased 2X12 baking pan.
10. Refrigerate
11. Pre-heat the oven to 110 degrees.
12. After 4 to 12 hours take the cold piddlin' out of the fridge, and put on the bottom shelf of the oven.
13. After another 4 to 12 hours, put the pan on the top shelf.
14. With the purple fork, constantly check the crust which should be forming. When the fork snaps, your dish is ready!

YIELD: 5, but why share?

ROYAL PURPLE VEGETABLE BISQUE

You will need an autoclave for this dish. You can rent one from your local autoclave dealer.

INGREDIENTS/UTENSILS

1- 2 x 6 chameleon
2 large grasshoppers
Chloroform
Purple construction paper
5 shot-glasses of blackberry brandy
4 medium sized purple potatoes
7 prunes.
More blackberry brandy
1 Autoclave
1 purple fork

INSTRUCTIONS:

1. Plug in the autoclave.
    An autoclave should never be left plugged in. Plug it in only when you are ready to use it.
2. Put your chameleon on the purple paper.
3. Drink the first shot of blackberry brandy.
4. When the chameleon is completely purple, pour the chloroform on the grasshoppers. This will put them to sleep
5. Give the chameleon it's last meal of the chloroformed grasshoppers.
6. When the chameleon is smiling, Brindle it in the chloroform.
7. Wait two minutes until the white of the chameleon's eyeballs can be seen.
8. Poke the chameleon with a purple fork. If it turns over with its legs straight out, it's ready.

9. Drink the second shot of blackberry brandy.

10. Skin the chameleon. Put the skin in a glass bowl. Set the chameleon innards aside. *They can be used in "Gore Stew".*

11. Pre-gest the potatoes.

12. When fully pre-gested, add to the glass bowl.

13. Paste the prunes, then add them to the bowl.

14. Turn the autoclave to stun for 15 minutes.

15. Drink the third shot of blackberry brandy.

16. When the autoclave alarm goes off, the mixture is ready.

17. Using the steel foundry gloves, remove the bowl from the autoclave. Let sit.

18. Drink the fourth and fifth shots of blackberry brandy.

19. What the heck, drink the rest of the brandy.

20. Lie down.

21. When you wake up, the mixture should be ready to eat, if not, then it's too late, and maybe call and order a pizza or something.

YIELD: A family of four, or one golden retriever. They'll eat anything and everything.

Glossary

AIOLI: *n.* AIOLI: Come on! "Aioli?" Four vowels and a consonant? It'sa made-up sauce by the saucy Rachel Ray, the Loki of the cooking world.

ALDENTE: *adj.* A way of cooking spaghetti that makes it too stiff to enjoy.

ANTITOXIN: *n.* A person or group that hates toxins. Or, possibly, and I'm not saying this is something that I'm going to be proud of, not in any way, shape, or font, but "Antitoxin" could possibly be…and I'm just throwing this out there,

A "poisonous female relative."

APERITIF: *n.* A smidgen of liquid aftper dinner.

BARDLE: *v.* Throwing ingredients into a bowl from a height of four feet or more.

BIAS, ON THE: *v.* A prejudice cutting of ingredients.

BIG BONED: *n.* An old wife's tale, like alchemy. It's not possible to turn metal into gold. It's also not possible for fat to turn to bone. Is it? I don't know, all the research isn't in yet, but who knows, "science" is discovering new diseases every day, so that ad agencies can put ads on TV singing their praises, but then very quickly at the end of the ad, tell you to not take the drug if you are allergic to it, which you wouldn't know until you took it, right? But fat to bone? I suppose if you are instantly baked in a lava flow like the people of Pompeii it could happen. By the by, the word "pompous" comes from that ill-fated island/nation. They were so sure the volcano would never blow, they were pompous about it.

BISQUE: *n.* A snappy/crispy form of soup. Enjoyed mainly by fashion models, and web site designers.

BLACKEN: *v.* The darkening of a mixture, whether you meant to do it or not. Note: Meats are not the only ingredient that can be blackened. Any ingredient can be blackened, but I wouldn't recommend it because it is irreversible.

BLANCH: *v.* What happens to your face when your soufflé falls. Also: A relative of STELLLLAHHHHH!

BLEND: *v.* A kinder, gentler form of mixing ingredients in to one homogeneous group. The mixing of ingredients until you can't tell where one ingredient starts and the other ends.

BOLOGNESE SAUCE: *n.* Sauce made from putting bologna through an orange juice squeezer.

BOMBE: The best dessert. "You are going to love this dessert, It's the Bombe!"

BORING KNIFE: *n.* A very dull knife, so be careful. It's used in a lot of films where the house person is being mugged by a mugger, as muggers are won't to do, and as they are being mugged, the house person reaches behind them and grabs the knife they left out on the counter and then stabs the mugger with it, which, since the knife is so short, only angers the mugger, and he or she then takes it out on the dog.

BOUILLON: *n.* A "moullion" times ten.

BOWLS: *n.* Round or square containers: Could be copper, plastic, metal, stainless steel, Teflon, super, orange, or rose colored.

BRINE: *n.* Salty wine. Delicious. Sort of a "ChardonYEA!"

BRAISE: *v.* Complementation of meat: "I took a piece of meat,and braised it to the heavens.

BRINDLE: *v.* The marinating of animals while they are still alive.

BUNDT: *v.* Moving food forward just a little.

CAN CLOSER: *n.* An implement used to cover previously opened cans. Also used to shut the bathroom door.

CAN OPENER: n. The person who has to go to the bathroom, or more formally, the "waste disposal facility".

CARMELIZE: *adj.* To take a nice trip up U.S. 101 the northern coast of California.

CHARLOTTE ROUSSE: *n.* The actress Charlotte Rae's recipe for angel food cake. Charlotte Rae, I'm pretty sure, is the Grand Aunt of Rachel.

CHARLOTTE MOUSSE: *n.* Ditto for the actress's chocolate dessert often seen on The Facts Of Life, where she brilliantly played Mrs. Garrett. CHARLOTTE MOUSSE also serves as a sweet hair gel.

CHARLOTTE GOOSE: *n.* One of the actress's gamier recipes.

CHARLOTTE VERNOOSE: Night time wear for the sexy star.

CHEESE CLOTH: *n* A cotton piece of cloth used to strain sauces and all things liquid. In ancient times, actually a sort of sieve made entirely out of goat's cheese that was flattened using a cheese press, then left out in the rain, dried, and voila,! there's your cheese cloth, In modern times it is made of cotton, or wool.

CHEESE PRESS: *n.* A utensil made to make cheeses thinner than thin, without breaking it. (The cheese. The press itself is pretty much indestructible. God knows I've tried.)

CHEWOLOGY: *n.* The science of crushing food by moving the jaw up, down, sideways, until the food is pre-gested.

CHOOF: *n.* A cook that is almost a chef. *V.* Blowing on food to CRESTLE it.

CLARIFY: *v.* Making sure you understand exactly what is needed in the recipe. The proper utensils to use, and the measuring instruments.

CLAY POT: *n.* It's a *pot*, made of *clay*. Also: It's what happened To Ali's abs when the boxer got old.

CLEAVER: *n.* Dangerous item used in old, corny movies that take place in the Orient. Also: Beaver.

CREAMER:*n.* Something to contain the cream and keep it from spilling all over the place: Also: The Green Bay Packers when playing The Chicago Bears.

CRESTLE: *v.* This is what happens when you blow on an ingredient or mixture at a 10° angle continuously for 30 seconds or more. A light crust should form on top of the ingredient or mixture.

CRESTLER: *n.* This funnel shaped instrument can cut crestling time in half.

CRIMP: *v.* Overhand stirring of food with the improper utensil causing a tiny muscle spasm in your stirring hand.

CRUDITE: *n.* A boorish food, or a person who eats with their mouth open.

CURE: *v.* Making food more delicious by aging it. Also, and I am absolutely sure of this, fixing the recipe when you have made a mistake. Like RayRay always says: "If you think you have made a mistake, you haven't, you've just created a new recipe!"

CUTTING BOARD: A flat wooden, or plastic thing used when you want to cut, dice, slice, or otherwise maim perfectly good ingredients because you don't want to scratch your table top or dull the knife. Also: a company's group of execs that can fire people.

DARDLE: *v.* To boil a liquid until it contains a greater percentage of water than was previously in the container. It's actually a very small amount and you'll need an autoclave, but it can be done if you know the ins and outs of dardling.

DASH: *n.* Smaller than a PINCH. Also, Elan, brio, flash, suaveness.

DAB: *n.* Basically a JOT, but only for creams and lotions. "A little dab will do ya."

DEEP FRY: *v.* Frying that saturates the entire ingredient, top to bottom, side to side, leaving nothing that a doctor would recommend eating, even though she or he eats it him or herself.

DILLDOUGH: n. Money used to buy kosher pickles.

DISOLVE: *V.* A melting of ingredients into puddles.

DISORIENT: *v.* Mixing the ingredients so fast that that it is impossible to tell one ingredient from the other.

DRIZZLE: *v.* A slight addition of an ingredient or ingredients either liquid or solid, animal, vegetable or mineral.

DUST: Less than even a DRIZZLE. The absolute minimum of ingredient. Done right, the other ingredients can be seen through the dust.

DUSTER: *n.* A utensil used to put a fine powder-like coating of a usually whitish ingredient on a recipe. *n.* What you should wear when giving food a coating of a dusty like material.

EGG TIMER: n. This is a device farmers use to make sure the eggs come out of their chickens just at the right time for freshness. Sometimes the eggs have to be manually pulled out of the chicken.

EMULSIFY: *v.* Making the food mixture smaller than the wart on a butterfly's fanny.

ENTREE: *n.* Entree is a French word, and like almost every single French word, it is spelled incorrectly, but that aside, in its application to gas*tronomy. The word itself, "ENTRÉE" is French for "On the Tray." It also means to come into a place; "Entree Vous", which is French for "You Enter". Related to food, it is an entering of the food into one's mouth. In the good 'ol U.S.A.! One of the few countries in the world that proudly makes sure only healthy people stay healthy, in finer restaurants*, "Entrée" means the main course.

    * "gas" is right if you've had partaken of French food. Frogs legs, crepes, pate, foie gras, poutine, and brie will all give you a good case of the trumpets.

    ** A restaurant with one page menus, and entrees that have at least 15 items you've never heard of

ENZYME: *n.* Newly discovered conglomeration of atoms, acids, and cosmic dust bunnies. Originally it was thought that enzymes. were basically bacteria with fewer legs.

EXTRACT: *v.* To take ingredients out of the cabinet or drawer. Also: *n.* The past tense of "tract."

FLANK: *v.* The butt of a meat. Also: *adj.* to flank. To make sure there are ingredients on all sides of the counter or table.

Fondle: *v.* A very gentle way of adding ingredients to a recipe.

FOOD PROCESSOR: A catalogue of illegal foods.

FLAB: *n.* An autological word (a word that sounds like it's definition.) especially if you say it slowly and over enunciate: "flaaaaabbbbb."

FLABBING: *v.* Chatting about your diet or someone else's lack of one. "The two guys were talking about their flabby beer bellies."

FLAN:*v.* Preparing to make a delicious kind of pudding. "I'm flanning a delicious dessert for dinner.

FOOD PROCESSOR: *n.* A highly dangerous device that can drastically change solid food into liquid food.

FORMAGGIO: *n.* Food for the greatest Yankee baseball player in history. Also: It's a type of cheese. (Personal opinion: "Cheese" should be spelled with a "z", not an "s", like it's counterparts: "Freeze!", "Wheeze" "Squeeze" and "Sneeze".)

FRESH: *adj.* Alive. Not dead.

FRICASEE: *n.* A dish of stewed or fried pieces of meat, in a white sauce. *V.* The Southernizing of any food.

FUDGE: *v.* Skimping on your ingredients. "I fudged on the flour a little bit."

FUSE: *v.* A permanent blending of ingredients. You will never, ever be able to separate them.

GANACHE: *adj.* Something that gives a French person that saucy quality, similar to the great Maurice Chevrolet, Jacques Brel, Catherine Deneuve, Marquise De Sade, Toulouse-Lautrec, Charles Aznavour, Napoleon, Yo-Yo Ma, Vincent van Gogh, Brigitte Bardot, Charles Boyer, King Louie Jourdan, and the quite insane, Edie Piaf.

GARNISH: *n.* Taking money out of one's wages for delinquent child support payments.

GINGER: *n.* Cookies. These delicious snaps were named after the delightful actress on Gilligan's Island.

GLOSSARY: *n.* A compilation of words that sometimes define or explain them.

GRATE: *n.* The thing that keeps food from becoming charred embers and somewhat inedible.. *V.* Excoriating food into small bits. *Adj.* What you want people to say after they eat your food.

GUMBO: *n.* Gumby's brother. Also, the sixth Marx Brother.

HERB: *n.* Invented by Marquis Herb de la Artoise, who ate nothing but spices. In less civilized countries, like England, it is pronounced with the "H" sound.

HOBNOB: *v.* Introducing the ingredients to each other before fusing or mixing them.

HORS D'OEUVRE: A crazy fun word to pronounce.

JOT: *n.* Basically a DAB, but thrown at the other ingredients, rather than just "added."

JULIENNE: *n.* My ex.

KNEAD: *v.* Massaging ingredients, not necessarily just dough. Anything can be kneaded, even vegetables, meats, and/or fish.

KNIFE SHARPENER: *n.* Tool to make knives sharp enough to cut the crap out of things including thumbs and fingers. Once I cut off the tips of two fingers, but I immediately put them in ice, and drove to the emergency room. Unfortunately, they put the wrong tip on the wrong finger and vice versa. No knows this, except my therapist. And now you.

KOSHER SALT: *n.* A very salty salt, that is blessed by a rabbi, even a reform rabbi.

KUSHER SALT: *n.* Salt that is 25% saltier than plain Kosher salt

KUPP: A dead news reporter

LAZY SUSAN: I'm not going to lower even *myself* for this one.

-LINI

    CREMINI: Pasta dish

    PORCINI: Pasta dish

    TORTILINI: Pasta dish.

    LINGUINI: Pasta dish

    THE GREAT SANTINI: Movie about pasta.

LOIN *n.* : A dirty word

MANGLE: A device that mixes the ingredients in a way they should be mixed, but renders them completely anonymous. Also, it is cruel to some ingredients, and will fight them in the mixture and in your stomach.

MATOZISE: *n. or v.* Don't know, but saw it in a recipe once.

MENDLE: *n.* A reckless folding of ingredients.

MINCE: *v.* A prissy movement like Poirot, the French Detective. Little known fact: Poirot was known in his inner circle for making cozy hats out of dinner leftovers.

MINGLE: *v.* The combining of ingredients for a short period of time. Usually between a hobnobbing, and blending.

MIX: Stirring ingredients into a bowl

MUDDLE: *v.* Slap-dash way to introduce ingredients in a bowl. Also: Calling an ingredient something other than its real name.

MEASURING FORK: *n.* Used instead of a MEASURING SPOON if you only want about 1/10th of the ingredient in the recipe.

MEASURING SPORK: *n.* Transgender utensil

MULL: *v.* Aging of ingredients until they will get people drunk.

NORD PAS de VALAISE *n.* Movements when adding Herbes de Provence or French wines to a recipe.

OBESE: *adj.* Very big, to the point of stretching the skin so far, that it sometimes splits and the innards spill out. You also can't see your genitals with a mirror. This term doesn't just apply to people. An idea can be OBESE. Objects may be OBESE. If an object is obese it can't fit on a table even with all three leaves in.

ORZO: *n.* About, or around

PARBOIL: *n.* An average heating of liquids.

PASTE: *v.* Hitting pizza dough a good one.

PINCH: *adj.* More than a JOT, or PINCH, but less than a DAB.

PINCHETTE: *adj.* Less than a PINCH, but more than a JOT, or a PINCH, about equal to half a SMIDGEON.

PIZZELLE IRON:*n.* Hahahahahahaha. But seriously, one can make pizzles with this device.

POUND CAKE: *n.* A delicious food that hardly ever weighs exactly a pound. It's also an insult: "Why don't you go pound cake buddy"

PREGEST: *v.* Chewing of food before serving it to guests.

PREJEST: v. The telling of a good joke to loosen up everyone before they eat, making it easier on the digestion process.

QUADRILLAGE: *v.* A military assault with four soldiers armed with bayonets only. It is also a combining of four ingredients at once.

REDUCE: *v.* To take an overage of ingredients out of the mix

REGEST: *v.* Opposite of ingest. Also known as "ralph", "chork", "heave", "barf", "hurl", "chunder", or "squeep."

RE-FUSING: *v.* If an ingredient is added too late to a recipe, there might be some unwanted separation of ingredients. If that happened, you would need to re-fuse them. or if done correctly, after an initial fusing, the ingredients become even harder to tell apart.

RELISH:*n.* Like it sounds: An addition to any recipe that adds something that makes you anticipate the deliciousness of the prepared food.

ROLLING PIN: *n.* This familiar item, is usually a wooden tool for which it is difficult to find space in a kitchen drawer. It is used for flattening ingredients.

ROUND ROLLING PIN: *n.* The ROLLING PIN that normal people use.

ROUX: French for chess pieces looking sort of like watchtowers in medieval times.

SCURDLE: *v.* Mixing ingredients in a heated pan with 1/2 inch of water in it. No more, no less.

SLITHER: *v.* Adding ingredients without them knowing

it. Usually done while casually whistling an innocuous tune.

SMIDGEON: *adj.* Much cuter than a PINCH.

SNIGGLE: *v.* Putting fewer ingredients in that are called for in the recipe.

SPRINKLE: *adj.* About a pinch, but dropped into the other ingredients in a very random movement.

SQUARE ROLLING PIN: *n.* For experienced chefs only. Used for fancy flattening.

SAGE: *n.* A herb. In lesser developed countries like England, it is actually pronounced like the guy. It got its name from a seer in the 1300's who ate only spices.

SAL DENTE: *n.* Al's Brother.

SAUTE: *n.* A city in southern France known for heavy grease.

SHRED: *v.* Shrek's Dad. No really, it means taking a solid ingredient and making it take up more space.

SIFT: *v.* Making some ingredients as small as they can get.

SIFTER: *n.* (SEE "SIFT")

SKIM: *v.* Taking something off the top.

SKIMP: *v.* Stingy form of skimming.

SIMMER: *n.* The really hot part of Summer

SNIFTER: *n.* Container for brandy to drink to make the cooking experience a happy one.

SNIGGLE *v.* Putting a silly ingredient in the mixture. Usually one that isn't in the recipe.

SPATULA: *n.* Flat rubber, plastic, or metal item for getting under food in a pan or other cooking devices.

SPITULA: *n.* Past tense of spatula.

STIFFEN: *v.* What you do if a guest spits out his food right after tasting it.

STRAINER: *n.* A person who is trying to lift a KitchenAidProfessional 60 Mixer™ out of the bottom shelf of a cabinet. There have been many injuries reported by people trying to do this. If they would have invested in an Oster product, they would not be wearing a back brace like they are now. Oster: "Professional quality, unprofessional slogans"

SUBSTITUTE: *v.* Switching ingredients, (as if the ingredients don't know it).

SUMMER SQUASH: A game played outside involving rackets, a ball, and walls.

SWINDLE: Taking some ingredients out of the mixture, or not adding something that should be added because you don't have it in your larder, or you can't afford it. Like pure lobster-casoury ($175 an ounce)

TEA OR TABLESPOON - HEAPING: *adj.* Enough ingredient to make a mound within the boundaries of the teaspoon. There should be a nice peak to the ingredient placed in the spoon without any spillage.

TEA OR TABLESPOON - LEVEL: *adj.* The ingredients in the spoon should perfectly fit within the boundaries of the spoon. You can make sure they are level with a SPOON SCRAPER (SEE, "UTENSILS") To make sure it is truly even, use a carpenter's level.

TENDERIZE:*v.* The softening of an ingredient to the point where they are much more lovable.

THIN: *v.* The weakening of a mixture and, for some screwed up reason, what you want to be.

TOFU PRESS: Utensil hoarded by hippies and vegetarians, vegans, and communists.

TOSS: *v.* Adding ingredients that are not mixed yet. Done by throwing the container up in the air, twirling it around, then, while holding the container, dancing to a Latin samba or the Charleston.

TWEAK: *n.* A PINCH with a twist.

TWEEKLE: Pre-tweaking of food.

VINAIGRETTE: *n.* A smaller amount of vinegar.

WAFFLE: *v.* Hesitating when putting in some ingredients in with what's already in the mixing bowl. Also, underestimating the CREEDBLES

WHISK: Using a whisker to whisk food. Difficult to use on solid ingredients.

WHIST: Twisting your whiskers while stirring the food.

WHIFFLE: *n.* Missing the bowl or container when adding ingredients.

WOK: *n.* An impressive utensil to use when guests are over, whether the recipe calls for it or not.

XERNOPHETE: *n.* Someone who is afraid of food, even though my spell-check denies it. Look it up.Or, a connoisseur of furry mammals as snacks.

YERBLE: *n.* Part rodent, part fish, mainly found in Wall S.D. Cultivated for its fleshy cheeks, and salty tail.

ZEST: Adding an Oooooowheeeee factor to your food.

ZESTER: *v.* An implement used to make your food to wake up and stand at attention.

Baseline Charts

WE'LL BE BACK AFTER THIS:
(Advertisement: You can skip this ad in 1/2 page]
ANNOUNCER: How many times has this happened to you?
It's 5 AM and the phone rings.
There's just muffled breathing on the other end.
You ask: "Who is this?!",

There's no answer, just the breathing, so you cup the phone and ask: "Ronald? Is that you? That's not funny Ronald, why are you calling on my house phone, when my husband is at home. There's no reply, just this awful, hoarse, breathing. You are just about to hang up when a woman's voice screams something in Gaelic into the phone, and hangs up. You are awake by now, so you get up, take off your pajamas, get a foot caught in a pant leg, stumble head first into the corner of the chiffarobe, or if you don't know how to spell that, the dresser, wipe up the blood with your pajama bottoms Go to the bathroom, look at the wound in your head, accidentally brush your teeth with tile caulk instead of toothpaste* step into the shower, turn on the water, scald yourself, jump out of the shower onto a bar of soap on the floor, slip, fall backwards hit your head on the faucet, which isn't one of those cheap plastic ones, but a special solid brass one that you just had installed the week before, and split the back of your head open. You lie unconscious on the floor until your oldest boy, looking for breakfast, finds you naked and bleeding on the floor.

(SKIP AD)

He can't turn away, thinks of taking pictures to put on social media, but does the right thing and calls 911. You end up in the hospital, head in a cast.

And suddenly it hits you: "What will I make for dinner?

Sound familiar? No? Doesn't matter. The fact remains, and most sane people believe, that when you had a day filled with bad juju, the last thing you want to do, is make dinner for a bunch of hungry kids, a philandering husband, and a teenage boy that has just seen you naked and bleeding on the bathroom floor.

Perk up, because we have something that will save your klutzy butt. Menu plans!

Instead of trying to figure out what you are going to scrapple together for your gang each night, sometimes at the last minute, every recipe in the Color Diet Book can be frozen and then defrosted the whenever you don't have the time to put together a meal that will correspond with the "COLOR OF THE DAY"™.

Simply write the day of the week and color on the package that will be frozen.

TIGHT SHOT. Our recipes are specially blended to actually taste better after being defrosted. Not only that, the more you freeze and defrost, freeze and defrost, the more flavor will be added to the meal. Sound impossible?

Yes it does. But if you told Edith Piaf when she was a child, that someday, we'd land on the moon, she would have said "en accuse facon!" There are so many things that at one point in time, no one believed would be possible. Lawyers advertising on TV? Impossible? Test tube babies? "Hello!" A fourteen- year- old as president? Happened.

So you see, before you pooh pooh the "freeze/defrost" theory of added flavor, let us sum it up in one ironic word: Viagra.

Who'da thought?
EAT COLOR!
(Back to the book):

ACTIVITY/CALORIES PER MINUTE (CPM)

There are many things you can do in a day, and some of them burn calories, some of them do the opposite, and some of them ruin lives, and wreak destruction in your trail. Unfortunately, the latter, burns up the most calories. As you will see in the following chart, "wreaking havoc" is number one in burning calories.

ACTIVITY	CPM
Babysitter - one kid	4,060
Babysitter – 2 kids under 6	6,504
Basketball (1/2 court)	135
Dating (Third base)	1,700
Basketball (full court)	270
Frolicking	285
Kissing	10
Kissing (French)	220
Madden Football	1
Panic Attack (per hour)	580
Sex (normal)	230
Sex (kinky)	1,299
Tackle Football (Full Game, Guard)	17,000
Wreaking havoc	300 to 100,000

WEIGHT/HEIGHT/GENDER NORMS (naked, recent bowel movement)

HEIGHT	FEMALE/WEIGHT	MALE/WEIGHT
3'2"	54	61
3'7"	60	75
4'1"	78	84
5'2"	110	127
5'6"	122	149
5'8"	150	150
5'10"	165	200
6'4"	179	200
6'8"	202	220
8'2"	301	500

Q & A

Questions will be indicated by the letter "Q" and Answers by the letter "A" unless a question is asked by the Answerer, or/and an answer is given by the Questioner, pretty much making the whole Q&A system a travesty.

FREQUENTLY ANSWERED QUESTIONS

Q: How much sleep should I get when I'm on this diet?

A: See the "SLEEP/WEIGHT/AGE/OCCUPATION CHART in our next book. It will tell you how much sleep you need according to your weight, age, and occupation. For instance, A 75 year old accountant who weighs 152 pounds, should get 6 hours and fifteen minutes of sleep a night or day.

Q: Will Molten Egg Pie give me the runs?

A: Depends.

Q: I have been on your Color Diet for 10 months now, and have lost

217 pounds. My problem is that I have a lot of sagging skin. What can I do?

A: With sagging skin, you will want to: Swing it to and fro, tie it in a knot, tie it in a bow, fling it over your shoulder, like a continental soldier, 'cause your skin hangs low.

Q: Is it feed a fever and starve a cold, or feed a cold and starve a fever?

A: What does this have to do with the Color Diet™?

Q: Nothing

A: In that case, it's steve a fold, and carve a steever.

Q: I am 80, should I jog?

A: Sure, why not, what do you have to lose? You're old, you might as well live on the edge. But in all seriousness, we don't care.

Q: How do I convince a friend to go on the Color Diet™?

A: You can't. You shouldn't. Why would you? What kind of friend are you, anyway? Implying your friend needs to lose weight or be healthier? We think you should go to a tact class. Do you think you are God's gift to the light and lively? Leave them alone. If God didn't want heavy sick people, he wouldn't have invented bariatric potty seats, or stomach stapling or Ju Ju bees. But if you insist on violating your roommate's body space, do this. Tell them you want to take their picture. When you point the camera at them, tell them to hold on because you have to get a wider angle lens to get all of them in the shot. Let them stew on that for a while.

Questions From Readers

Q: Hi, I'm RED CUTSAP, from Dust Texas, and I luuuuve to barbecue. Does that fit in with this "color" thing?

A: Yes it does Red.

Q: What?

A: I said yes it does, Red.

Q: Ok, I heard that, I meant what effect does it have on the diet.

A: Oh. Well, first let's ask the question: Does BBQ-ing have anything to do with colors of food in the Color Diet. The answer is basically no. But beyond that, yes, of course it does. Red, I hate to tell you this, because as a Texan, you love your barbecue, Right?

RED: Right I shurrrrrrrr do.

A: ...I bet....and I dare say, if your house was on fire, and you had to choose between saving your wife or your back porch barbecue grill, I think we all know how that would turn out.

RED: Yep.

A: You would make a mad dash into the house, pull out a few steaks from the freezer, right?

RED: Yup.

A: And use the fire to grill them for dinner for a few of your hunting buddies. Right?

RED: Yup.

A: Disappointing news Red, not only is smoke from Barbecue fires the major cause of pollution in Texas, charring meat gives off compounds called heterocyclic amines, which cause cancer in laboratory animals exposed to them, which is why laboratory animals never barbecue, nor should laboratory animals *be* barbecued But it does beg the question: When the laboratory scientists barbecue meat for these tests, do they just blow the smoke in the test animals' faces or do they feed the barbecued meat to the little animals to whom they are giving cancer? And of course, we also have to ask about polycyclic aromatic hydrocarbons and what they do to the ozone layer.

In Canada, according to the Canadian Department of Justice, charcoal is now a restricted product under the Hazardous Products Act. Finally, propane vs coals: The National Anti-Propane industry states that: "Injury and death can result from the improper use of propane, and being aware of potential dangers associated with the volatile gas could save lives."

RED: Whoa Nelly! That's frickin' insane.

A: Yup.

Nettie Frothwattle, Northumberton Chelsea, United Kingdom.

Q: Why isn't there a blue food group?

A: Interesting question. Here's an interesting answer: There are almost no blue foods, therefore, they are wrapped neatly into the Purple category. I mean, "blueberries" are supposedly "blue", but if you put them on a true-blue cardigan sweater for instance, they don't look blue at all. They look purple. Blueberries are actually purple.

A: Let me give you an analogy. The structure of an atom, is like a solar system. The nucleus is its sun, and the electrons are the planets revolving around them, their sun.

Q: What does that have to do with food groups?

A: Nothing, but it's a good analogy, isn't it? If we were to make things up in this manual, we would say that the analogy is that food is the sun, and the colors of the food are the electrons revolving around their sun.

Don't be fooled by stereotypes. Is all asparagus green? No! Are all carrots orange? No siree bob tail cat they aren't. Are all tomatoes red? You'd have to be born in a bath tub to think that they are. Are all Lemons yellow? Yes. They are, so never mind.

Neil Stevehat, Buxom MO.

Q: I'm Neil Stevehat, from Buxom MO. What about beef. If it's rare, isn't it red in the middle?

A: Well, Mr. Stevehat, if you don't mind us calling you that, we use the C.I.U.I. I. test. Mr. Stevehat (It appears you like to have your name repeated as much as possible) "Cook It Until It's Inedible". So in the case of your beef, cook it until no one would want to eat it, and you will find that it is brown.

Dickie Muttleknob, Shelves IA.

Q: What about liver, it's kind of red.

A: Yes it is. But if you cook it until it's inedible, it'll be ok.

Q: How do you eat something that's "inedible"?

A: Obviously you've never been really hungry, or had dinner at my Aunt Eileen's house. And I think you're referring to the term: *Un*edible. There's a huge difference.

Barca Rajgeeka: Condorville, Tunk.

Q: What about Brussels sprouts. They turn brown when you cook them.

Q: Are you sauteing them?

A: Yes.

A: Don't do that.

And I hope to your god, that you are not using butter. Unless, you pan fry the butter until it is brown. If you don't brown it, that's adding yellow to a green, and that would defeat the purpose of the Color Diet

Captain Helton Git: A Submarine somewhere in the North Sea. But maybe not. It may be in the Red Sea, or just off of Cape Cod. Who knows? Not us, that's for certain, so don't ask, if you found out, we'd have to torpedo you.

Q: What if a food is partially another color?

A: Well, Sir, that might happen, but here's the solution:

Go with the 98% Rule. Take lettuce. I mean pay for lettuce. If 98% of the color of a head of lettuce is green, it's ok to eat the whole thing. But if you'd be eating only 85% green and 15% white, just eat the green part.

Q: What about Cucumbers? They are green on the outside and white on the inside.

A: Holy snotwipe, Captain, just peel the freakin' dark green. But furthermore, the inside of the cucumber, if you put it on the Color Grading Scale device (Coloreter) you'll see the inside, is actually a pale pale matuse. Or light green.

Q: I have questions about lot's of other foods, you see…here on a submarine, we have limited…

A: Sorry for interrupting, Capt'n but I heard the "smoke 'em if you got 'em" whistle…got to go. Before I do, I have a question for you: Did anyone on your submarine, every climb into the torpedo tube thingy, and accidentally get shot out? They do it in the circus, I figured they could do it in the navy.

Q: Yes, happens all the time.

Shaunagain Doggledannie, Loch Bealach a' Mayonaise, Scotland, U.K.

Q: I'm kind of heavy, but I hardly eat anything. Just a few bites a day, but I still can't lose any weight. Suggestions?

A: Yeah, sure. "You are *kind of* heavy, and only eat a "few bites a day?" Yes, and Hitler was just in a bad mood, Madonna actually is a virgin, the check is in the mail, I'll respect you in the morning, I've tried to be nice to my husband, and it's safe to walk anywhere in New York now. Nice try Shaun.

Fodor Miskowitz, Sleepover, Camp.

Q: What about nuts, like Brazil nuts? They are brown on the outside, but white on the inside. Do we have to shave off the brown skin, or whatever it's called.

A: It's called the pellicle, and in the "Bible of Color In Food", written by a guy named William Sonoma, who was basically the William Shakespeare of food, wrote, in his brown chapter, one of the catagories is nuts. Practically every nut you can think of is listed in this Brown Category. The brown skin is hard to get off, but it can be done with a solution of Ammonia, vinegar, and melted X-lax ™ tablets. But I would go with William S. He seems to know what he is talking about. Most of the time. Except when he groups "blue" in the Purple/Red category.

MORE A&Q

Selene Selene, Moonpie MO

Q. Why is this a separate section of questions? Why not just continue with the Q & A in the paragraph above?

A. First of all, they aren't in a "paragraph". It's more of a "section".

Second of all, why do you have the same first and last name? Why don't you just include the two names into one?

Third of all, it's our book, and we can do whatever we want.

Fourth of all, this section is "A&Q" and if you were paying attention, the first section was "Q&A

Fifth of all, it adds "bulk" to the book, which is important to the whole publishing process, A book without "bulk" is basically a pamphlet.

EVEN MORE QUESTIONS AND ANSWERS (just to spite Selene Selene)

Frau Astrid von Buchenwaldermunch, Sthadenhauser East Germany

Vy should ve trust you, Mister "Chudnow" if that's really your name, vat creditability do you have for this?

A: Good question Frau, Buchenwaldermunch, why indeed should you trust me?

Q: Vat?

A: I said, why should you?

Q: Louder!

A: I said: there's no reason to, Frau Buchenwalermunch!

Q: LOUDER!!

A: I SAID YOU DON'T HAVE TO TRUST ME!

Q: DON'T YELL AT ME, SWINEHUNT!

A: Ok, Sorry, but seriously, you do bring up a very good question. Why trust us? Who are we to suggest a health-filled diet plan? We are just scientists, researchers, and food technicians. We are only the dedicated Mother Teresas of food, who studied food, and its ins and outs for years, probably since you were a big deal in the Bundestadt. We are People, Frau Buchenwaldermunch, people who have devoted our lives to this mystery of this so called "food" and what part it can play in people's lives. We who have basically ignored our families, our friends and normal lives, to unlock these mysteries. Why should you trust us, indeed! I say, Harrumph, Frau Buchenwaldermunch!

You can't face the food, Buchenwaldersthein!! You, atop your Bavarian Castle tower, munching your Strudelvort, thinking that you can ask anything you want, in that haughty, snide, guttural, grunt you call Chermin, and then expect to get an answer from us, us, who haven't inherited anything, but worked our fingers to the bone, experimenting on our own bodies, endangering, and sometimes sacrificing our very lives so you, you piece of semmelknuedel schnitzel, can live longer and better! We all hope you choke on a large piece of Spaetzel Wurstkuchen, Buchenwaldermunch,

So, thank you, and enjoy swimming in your crocodile infested moat.

Sandra Schlopsky: Fort Knuck, Cloud Nine, Wisconsin:

Q: Who was that insane lady?

A: That was my Aunt Heidi.

Dusty Roads, Kantchasink, Sixinch Poland:

Q: Can we still go on eating even if we are full? (As long as it's the right color, of course).

A: That full feeling that you are talking about Dusty, is your body telling you that you have to stop eating until you poop some of the food out, to make room for more. I know some people who have given themselves enemas so they could go on eating. Normally I don't recommend that, but this is a semi-free country, so go ahead. Just do it in the privacy of your own home.

Arthur Bill Stevens, Suicide Falls, S.D.

Q: I have been on the diet for two months now, and my waist and hips have shrunk, but my breasts have gotten larger!!

A: Good?

Melba Sowitalitty, Candou, France

Q: What if I forget the rotation schedule, and I eat green food on my yellow day?

A: Ok, here's what you do. The next day, eat the color food that you missed, so that the two are just reversed that week, then keep the same schedule the next week. Wait, that won't work. Ok, here's what you do. Skip a day, then start all over with a new rotation. Wait. No. Don't do that. Ok...ok...um.... here's what you do....you wait until I figure this out and get back to you, so sit tight, and don't eat anything until I do.

Bustar Hymann, Cowpie, Alabama.

Q: Can you smoke while on the Color Diet™?

A: Did you mean, "may" I smoke?

Q: Yeah, whatever dude.

A: No need to be rude Mr. Hyman.

Q: Yeah, yeah, just give me a frickin' yes or no answer, ok? Geezus, frickin' Christ! I don't have time for bulltwaddle.

A: Oh, ok. Of course. Of course you need an answer, and you need it fast. I understand that, and I'm guessing that you sound out of sorts because you are out of cigarettes. So what's the answer?

Let me tell you a little story, it won't take much of your time, but I think it would be important for you to listen. I know that it helped me in my time of angst.

Q: Ok, just make it quick, dude.

A: I will make it as terse as possible. "Terse" means "short"

Q: Holy shitstack, GET ON WITH IT!

A: Of course, Mr. Hyman. It seems that there was this army PFC (that stands for Private First Class…which makes one wonder if there is a private "second" or "third" class. But "First Class" sounds cool, doesn't it? Like if your kid is taking advanced logic classes in high school, or all college prep classes…..)

Q: Grrrrrrrrrr

A: So this PFC, never smoked in his life. He was only 22, so he had plenty of time to pick up the habit, and…. "habit" is an interesting word, isn't it? It could mean clothing, like a Nun's habit, or a costume worn for horseback riding, or bodily appearance, like a "fleshy" habit, sometimes it means the prevailing disposition or character of a person's thoughts and feelings, as in: that guy is always an impatient ass, or the mental make up a philosophical habit, I think it also could mean a behavior pattern acquired by frequent repetition or physiologic exposure that shows itself in regularity or increased repetition, say, when someone is always a bloated jerk that not even a grandmother could like…… so many meanings….

Q: DUDE!….

A: Oh, sorry… One night, our PFC, let's call him "Joe" (we won't reveal his real name, which is definitely not "Joe"), goes to a USO show. Now the USO, as you well know, as we all well know, is a wonderful magnanimous organization, one that entertains, and otherwise delights our boys, girls, and possibly transgenders in uniform with jolly amusements, and diversions, to keep our boys in the khaki from having to think about the possibility of hand to hand combat, where they might have to gut the enemy, while said snakes in the grass, are looking them directly in the eye or worse, both eyes, with a look that says: "Mommy!"

This PFC, this not-Joe, was at a USO show, you know the kind where the generals don women's clothes and dance and sing….it's hysterical…and while this is going on the guy next to "Joe" or some other name, our PFC, offered him a cigarette. Now, here's the important part, the reason I started this story in the first place. This man. Our PFC said "no, I don't smoke," so he didn't accept one. Then this other guy, let's call him "Jim" told him that he's lucky he didn't have vices, but Joe, says: "I'm not saying I don't have any vices," and Jim says: "oh really, and Joe, said yes, and Jim said what vices do you have, and Joe said "none". And Jim said "really?", and Joe says: "That's right, you know why I don't have any vices"? And Jim replies: "no I don't, Jim, amazed, asks: don't you have any vices?" Whereupon, Joe says: "I don't have any vices, because I don't call my Didoes vices, instead, I call them "activities." Then Jim goes, "oh", I get it, like the Socratic platitude, as he was instructing Plato in the vomitarium of the Coliseum, right?

Yes," says Joe, "exactly!" Thereupon, they became close friends, and revealed everything to each other, which eventually led to "Joe" becoming Jodene. The two eventually married, and now live in Compton with their two lovely adopted Applalachian children.

Q: And…..?

A. So you can smoke. Just use brown cigarette paper. And try and be nicer, and maybe finally come out to your family. It's not so….

Q: Ass. (click)

A: You're welcome, think nothing of it my man-woman, it's what we do.

From Our Hotline

Q: Can *anyone* do this diet?

A: Yes.

Q: Who?

A: Anyone, and everyone.

Q: But what people specifically shouldn't do this diet?

A: Ok, if you insist, If anyone shouldn't do this diet, it would be sports agents.

Q: What about alcohol, cigarettes and caffeine?

A: What about them? Don't smoke after a green salad because cigarette tobacco is brown, And don't have Lutefisk after drinking red wine. By the way, did you know that Madison, MN is called the Lutefisk capital of Minnesota?

A: No, I didn't.

Q: What about exercise?

A: What about it?

Q: Should we still exercise?

A: No. Exercise may just be the devil in disguise. You will never need to do one scoach of exercise while on this diet. Proper enzyme digestion tightens the quads, hardens the pecs, builds up the lats, encourages the biceps, and generally eats up the calories. Warning: If you quit the diet in the following week, you will gain all the fat back you used to have, and you will lose all muscle tone."

Q: I like being "fat". Anything wrong with that?

A: As we stated earlier, we love the adiposed people as we would love our own children, even if our children were to be lardy as a Texan oil magnate. Or any Texan for that matter. Be as immense as you want! But…don't feel bad when you can't get a job, romance, or are turned away at all you can eat buffets.

Q: Why is it called "The Color Diet?"

A: I'm not going to dignify that question by answering it.

(Crap, I just did)

(Oh well, too late to erase it now)

Q: I have been on The Color Diet™ for two months now. I have stuck to your instructions religiously and have lost two pounds. Now here's the weird part, I am throwing up 15-20 times a day, and have broken out in orange pustules all over my body, I have a temperature of 106, haven't slept in six days, and all my curly, beautiful hair is falling out in handfuls. There are blisters on my toenails, and I have shrunken tongue syndrome. What should I do? Please help me!!

Johnny Depp, Hollywood CA

A: Are you *the* Johnny Depp, the movie star? Holy cow! Johnny Depp, the famous movie star, is actually on the Color Diet™! Wait until I tell everyone! Ha! Wow

Q: I love your diet book. So creative, so helpful, genius work. Everybody loves it. I keep it on my kitchen counter, right next to the pictures of our three wonderful children.

A: Thanks Mom.

Q: Do you talk to your Sister?

A: Of course.

Q: Good, Family is more important than anything. Except health.

A: Gotta go, Ma, writing a book.

Q: You go, you write, I'll be here right by the phone when you finish your big important book.

A: (Sigh)

Testimonials

Dear Diet Tribe:

I assumed your diet book about foods and color was a big hoax, but then again, I thought the moon landing, having to drink eight glasses of water a day, and male pattern baldness were big hoaxes too. I also thought my cousin would move out after three months like he promised he would, but he didn't. Even after I dropped hint after hint he said he would, "as soon as I get a job". I even put plastic over his toilet seat, and put wintergreen in his jockstrap. Nothing worked. I'm not sure why my wife didn't back me up on this, but she seemed perfectly happy having him in the house while I went to work. "I feel safer" she said. Anyway, if you ask me, I think that your next book should be about how to remove people from your house, even if they are family. That's all. Thanks.

Donny "BigTime Graziano". Mainard, Maine

Dear Diet People:

I used to weigh 420 pounds. Now I only weigh 380, thanks to your flab-u-less Color Diet.

Fern Blofedelt, SoNo Chow, China

Diet People:

I heard about the Color Diet, I thought it was a joke. But I bought it for a laugh, and by the time I had finished reading it, I had lost three pounds, and *that's* no joke.

Neil Slickgnard, Plybar MN.

Sirs and Madames:
I had a headache, now I don't.

Sted Felmmchuckskorj, Netherlands.

Hi. I wrote you a while back about my Brother living in my house? Well, I took care of it. If you know what I mean. I have a house to myself now, I'm losing weight, and loving it. Thanks Color Diet.

Donny, Big Time Graziano, Witness Protection Program.
Ozaukee, WI.

Dear People Who Write Things:
I enjoyed your article on the rubber band. I collect them, and it was delightful, and life affirming to knows there is a club I can join that is full of people just like….wait…what? This isn't Latex Review? Sorry. PLEASE DON'T PRINT THIS LETTER.

Jeremy Codswallop, Piffle, Old Brunswick

Addendumb II

TIPS FROM THE PROS

Professional eaters, members of AEA (American Eaters Association), in their updated manual* on eating food and other things, "HOW TO EAT LIKE A PRO", have over a hundred valuable tips on ingestion. I have stolen what I thought were three that were the most valuable to any diet, and put them in my own words.

*There is a Spanish version of their manuel.

Here are the three pieces of advice:

1. D.E.A.D (Don't Eat Anything Dead)

"Fresh" fish! "Fresh" vegetables! "Just picked". You've seen the signs, you've heard the claims.

Let us set you straight. Forget everything you know about the word "fresh." Allow me to lift the "fresh" veil from your eyes. Is "fresh" really the best you can get? Let me tell you, my diet posse, that "fresh" is a mess of hooey, and I don't mean the whoooowheeee that is the yell so popular now amongst college kids drinking beer from funnels.

But how could everyone, except me, be so taken in by this "fresh is best" chicanery. Ok, ok, I know what you're are thinking: "does the bookstore accept returns without a receipt"? Look, I'm not saying that fresh isn't good, it is, but it's not the *best* you can do for your body, Even though the COLOR DIET doesn't have a list of foods you can eat while still on the vine, or the hoof, we just wanted to throw this out there. There is better than "fresh!"

"WHAT?" You say? 'How can that be? I don't understand. It sounds like a half-baked idea to me"

"Ha ha ho!" I say, gently mocking your naivety and your humor, because it's not your fault. Allow me to explain.

There is something that "fresh" "day old" or "stale" all have in common. Do you know what that commonality is?

READER: No, I don't.

ME: "Fresh", "day old", and "stale" are basically the same because even though something may be just picked, or only a day old, it is still...... dead!

READER: Yeah, so?

ME: Ok, it's time for you to zip it Betty Boop.

Everything you eat is dead.

There is only one way that a food is "fresh."

It has to be "alive" which means, the only vegetables that are "fresh" are the ones still on the vine. As soon as that tomato is picked it starts to lose its nutritional value. And worse, that value declines at a rapid pace. By the time it gets picked, packaged, put in the truck, driven to the supermarket, falls on the floor, and is put back into the bin, it has lost almost 50% of its nutritional robustness. Some grapes have a label admitting that they actually came from half way across the globe, or even further. Sometimes the food you finally get had been frozen, or on a boat, on rough seas, or on a truck on a bumpy road.

Do you truly think that these vittles, these comestibles that may have been tossed around like a kite in the wind, can possibly be "fresh"? No, you don't, and if you do, you shouldn't because you would be robbing yourself, and perhaps your family of all the nutritious fresh-osity they would otherwise get from food that is eaten while it's *still* on the vine, tree, or hoof."

Alive is best. Alive = Fresh, and conversely, Fresh = Alive. And if fresh = best, and alive = fresh, then alive = best. And mathematically, If fresh = alive, and if alive = backwards,≥ Dead+evila - afesh,= flive ÷-vile fish.≠Vail,÷ SERF = EVIL. So,.don't be fooled by random terminology.

READER: Mr. Chudnow, I don't get…

ME: Bitljnoiebububblebub! And call me "Sir"

READER: Sorry?

ME: Nothing.

READER: I was saying…..

ME: Gluppooltylnert!

READER: Forget…..

ME: Sherbidoodlebutt!

YOU: ….it.

ME: Ok, thanks.

If you can eat that apple before you pick it, if you can catch a fish with your teeth and eat it while it's in the water, or at least while it's still flopping around on land or in your skiff, you are eating fresh. If you can step up to a steer, and take a chunk out of its hide before it gets gruesomely, and inhumanly slain, you get every single juicy, nutrient filled morsel Mother Nature had intended for you, her special children.

Why do we cling to the theory that we have to kill something before we eat it? It's an ancient superstition, one that should be put aside along with walking under a ladder, breaking a mirror, and/or calling someone between 1:00 and 5:00 AM.

If you think that pre-historic man and /or prehistoric woman had weapons to kill its prey, you are sorely lacking in the sense we call common. Eventually, of course, they did have weapons, but in the Pre-Weaponical Age, they would just catch things with their hands, and eat whatever they had caught, raw. They would tear the flesh with their freakily sharp prehistoric saber toothed teeth. And when you think about it, like I am now, it's a great way to not deplete a food supply. The steer or horse heals, leaving 95% of it alive, and available for future breakfasts, lunches, dinners, or late- night snacks because an animal that is still alive has less chance of going bad.

It also has been proven far beyond a shadow of a doubt, in fact, literally in the brilliant sunshine of doubt, that the Pre-historics were healthier than we are now. Even healthier than that guy who skis, jogs, eats "pro-biotic" crap from huge containers from GNC, and never masturbates with his own hand. Yes, even healthier than Jane Fonda, workout version II. Why? Well, in those early days of man, not only did they eat it raw, they never cooked anything, because fire and crock-pots hadn't been discovered yet.

I think that we all know that cooking anything depletes it of most of its nutritional molecules.

And lastly, what about the animals we superior beings, us noble humans eat?

1. Fact! Animals have always been healthier than us, their human, and supposedly smarter counterparts.
2. Fact! Animals don't cook, steam, saute, scramble, parboil, roast, stew, or otherwise molest their meals.
3. Fact! Almost everything they eat is alive, or was alive moments before they killed it.
4. Fact! They never get gout, asthma, or piles.

You may now feel a little foolish cooking your food. So "GO RAW! "Raw raw raw, that's the spirit her at Color Diet U.

Gnaw away. You will love your body and your body will love you.

2. THE ART OF CHEWING

Chew..chew…chew…chew…chewchew….chuwchuwchuw-chew…Woooowhoooo, get on the mastication express! Next stop: Digestion!

Besides the color or pattern of your china, and the length of your silverware, chewing is the most important step, or link in the "eating chain" of the digestion continuum.

Here's a helpful tip from the top.*

Chewologists over the world, advise that before swallowing, chew each mouthful of food 100 times (the same amount, coincidently, that one should brush one's hair) on each side of the mouth. Then, they advise, take the lump of food out, drop it onto the plate, bowl, or whatever other means of pre-delivery you are using, look at it. Stare at it. Think about what lies there. Does it look like….fat? Then, after this revelation, play around with it. Roll it around with your utensil. Squish it, pat it, think of yourself as an artist, the food as your medium, and the plate as your palette. By now, you know the taste is gone, so why put it back in your mouth?

Almost anyone can swallow*, but mastering "the art the chew" will double your thinness in the blink of a bat's eye.***

We think that when you are done reading this book, you will double your thinness, and be as hot, and sharp as a waddle sandwich.

I don't know about you, but I'm feeling thinner already.

*The "top" is always "the best". The mountain top. The top of your class. The tips of asparagus, which is the only really delicious part of that venerable vegetable, the rest of the vegetable is basically part of the asparagus root system.

**Unfortunately some people *are* on feeding tubes. But even if they are, they can still observe the Color Diet™ regimen.

***Bats are the fastest blinkers in the animal kingdom.

3. PATTY CAKE PATTY CAKE - PLAYING WITH YOUR FOOD.

We've been told from the time we were able to put stuff in our mouths that we shouldn't play with our food. "Don't play with your food!" our collective mothers would yell at us. so we stopped playing with our food. The school of thought that told us we would I we just thought about sex, we would grow warts on our brains, or that if you cross your eyes, they will stay that way, is the same school of thought that told us to never play with your food. It is also the same school that would knock the crap out of your knuckles if you pulled Suzie Pritzkow's pig tails in third grade at Mt. Saint Helen's Catholic School for the Short.

Not playing with your food, has taken some of the joy of eating away from us. Us, who we love so dearly.

There is the "Joy of Cooking" cookbook. The "Joy of Growing Your Own Food" article in a magazine in a doctor's office somewhere, but why, oh God, why is there not a "The Joy of Playing With Food" manual?

It's true that there is *some* playing with our food. When we knead bread dough, or pie, or muffin , or whatever else is made from dough, we are basically playing with our food.

True story: At dinner, when we would have over-cooked hamburger, over boiled peas, and schmaltzy mashed potatoes, my Father would take his peas, mix them with his mashed potatoes, then squash his hamburger, add that to the potatoes and peas, then shape it into a big square, like a big box hardware store, and eat it one forkful at a time. He would chip away at the structure until there was just the loading dock left. My father was playing with his food! We would look on in fascination as he did this, and we were so proud to call him Ben."

Remember that food fight you had in high school cafeteria? Was not that just about the most fun you have ever had? It's hard to forget those all out, spontaneous, playful, sometimes painful meatball missiles, broccoli bombs, and ravioli rockets. They were pure flights of fancy food.

If you don't laugh when Curly gets hit in the face with a pie thrown by Larry, or when spaghetti is dumped on Moe's head, you need some intensive psychotherapy.

Come on, you've laughed at the meme of the kid who gets chocolate all over his face, hands, legs, clothes, high chair, floor, and walls, right? Of course you have. That's one of the things that is so wonderful about this "food" we have at our disposal. (No pun intended, but I'm certainly going to leave it in) Not only does food keep us alive, it keeps us laughing, and laughter is one of the roads to health.

I, myself, along with my best friend and cousin Lois, used to roll our mashed potatoes into little balls, and throw them at each other under the table at dinner, and laugh until we cried....from the spanking we got from Uncle Murray when he caught us doing it. The joy of food play has been systemically beat out of us like a dusty rug on a pioneer's porch.

Let's look at some of the fun games and exercises you can do to keep the play in your food.

Exercises and Games

TANGERINE JUGGLING

Tangerines are basically soft oranges. They aren't as round, but they are lighter. They are the perfect weight, shape and size for juggling.

The beauty of the tangerine, is that it is the fruit complement of actual juggling balls, or hacky sacks if you will, and even if you won't, they are perfect juggling material.

1. If you can't juggle, just start with two in one hand, throw one up, and catch it in the other. Do this over, and over, over, and over until you get the feel for it,
2. Upload the video: "How To Juggle"
3. Begin juggling.
4. When the peels are about to fall off, eat the tangerines,

PIZZA DOUGH FRIZBEE

1. Any number of teams. Two on a team.
2. The two players in each team start by standing about a foot from each other.

3. Each team starts with a ball of dough (each team has exactly the same size ball)

4. At the signal (yodel) The teams begin tossing the pizza dough back and forth between the two members of their team.

5. Each time they toss it, they take a giant step backwards. As the ball of dough is thrown, it should get thinner and thinner.

6. When it's thin enough to be made into a pizza, the team goes to a nearby store, gets ingredients, put them on the dough, and bakes the pizza in an oven.

7. The judges decide whose pizza is best. The pizzas are judged on:

   A. Which team is first to finish the pizza and present it to the judges. 15 pts.

   B. The quality of the ingredient. 10 pts.

   C. The thinness of the crust. 10 pts

   D. The overall taste of the pizza. 15 pts

ULTIMATE EGG TOSS

1. You will need 50 or 60 raw eggs.
2. Two teams of players stand about 50 yards apart.
3. Basically, it's a free for all.
4. Players pick up an egg and throw it at the other team.
5. Repeat until both teams are out of eggs.
6. There is no winner or loser.
7. The game ends in about 3 minutes.

HEADS UP TOSS

Ingredients:

Raw Eggs

Rules:

1. Each team has a tosser, and a catcher.
2. The catcher wears a construction helmet.
3. One team goes first.
4. Again, the Tosser and Catcher stand about 30 yards apart.
5. The first tosser, throws the raw egg high in the air.
6. It's the catcher's job to catch the egg on the top of his or her helmet.
7. Then the other team takes a turn.
8. A point is scored for each direct hit on top of the helmet.

FRISKY BEAN GAMES

"FRISKY BEANS" is a recipe found in the "RECIPE" section of this book,
It uses Mexican jumping beans and hot sauce.

BEAN CHOMP

To play:
1. The plate with the beans should be placed in the middle of the table, with each player equidistant from the plate.
2. Put all the hot sauce you have (at least a bottle), onto the beans, and then stand or sit around the plate of beans. Soon the hot sauce will cause the beans to do what they were born to do. Jump.

3. Without using your hands, try and capture the beans with your mouth while the beans are still in the air.
4. Set a kitchen timer for 2 minutes.
5. Whoever catches the most beans in whatever time limit you set, wins.

FRISKY BEAN HOME RUN DERBY

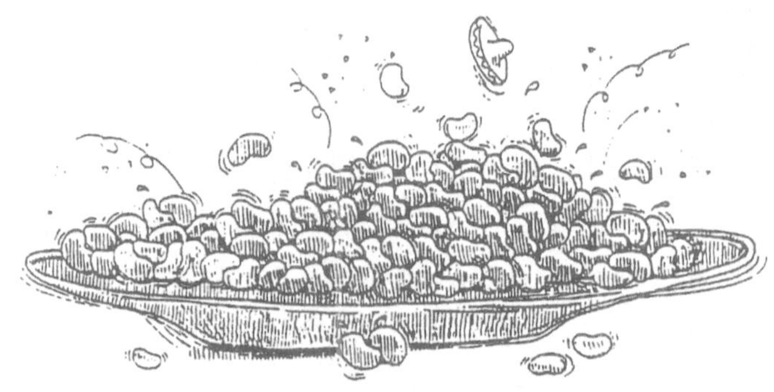

1. Follow the instructions for "BEAN CHOMP" but for this game you will need some sort of little bats, and separate plates. Butter knives would do nicely, or popsicle sticks. If tongue depressors are available, use those, they make the best bats for Frisky Bean Home Run Derby.
2. Set any kind of "Home Run Fence" up. It should be around 20 feet from the plate.
3. Using an indelible magic marker, mark the beans with a different color for each player.
4. Each player gets 30 seconds in the box to see how many of the beans on his plate he or she can knock out of the park.
5. If you are into competition (which I can't imagine not being into if you are playing this game), each player can find his or her own kind of hot sauce.
6. Think of it as race car teams trying to develop the more powerful engine.

EATING CONTESTS

Eating contests come in endless varieties of sizes, shapes, and flavors. We mention just a few of the contestial ingredients, after that, it's up to the participants' imaginations.

Obviously, there are several methods that are fun, and a number of foods with various degrees of difficulty that can be used for eating contests.

There is always the standard pie eating contest, the watermelon eating contest, and/or corn meal mush eating contest. But there are an infinite number of variations, some using your hands, some just your mouth Some include tossing the food item over a net before you catch it with your mouth. Here are a few.

1. *Pistachio Eating Contest.* You have to shell the nut with your teeth before you eat the meat. The shell is spit out toward a goal (similar to a dart board) and wherever the seeds land, the points are tallied, and counted toward the totals.

2. *Noodle-Sucking Contest.* The spaghetti noodles can't be grabbed with your teeth, they have to be sucked up one or two or three at a time.

3. *Face Licking Competition.* The competitors' faces are slathered in sauce, or some other viscous fluid. The contest involves trying to lick the substance off the other person's face so that the face is totally clean. The judges will judge the cleanliness of the face, including the ear holes and the nostrils. There is no time limit to this game.

4. *Banana peel and eat.* The bananas are put in a trough. Competitors must peel the banana with their teeth, eat the whole banana, then, just with the mouth, carry the peel to a teammate standing about 25 yards away, and then the teammate must carry the banana, peeled, with her or his teeth and deposit it into a garbage can another 25 feet away. The bananas can be all sizes or ply.

Bibliography

The King Jame's version of a Bible: Author: King James
The Koran: Author: Muhammed's friends.
"Confucious Say…": Author: Confucious
 "200 Positions for Pleasurable Eating" The Bhagaad Gita
"Politically Correct Recipes" Paula Dean
"Food Is Just a Four Letter Word" Author: Erich Segal
"Don't Bogart That Food" Author: Haile Selassie
"Everything You Wanted to Know About Food, And Were Afraid To Eat". Author: Ann Eorexic

Footnotes

*I have a small bunion on the big toe of my right foot.

*I never was into feet. I think they are pretty, for lack of a better term, hideous. These stubs coming out of a larger mass of skin, bone, and muscle?

*My toes are kind of clubby.

*My feet do not smell.

*I wear a size 81/2 tennis shoe, and a 9 in a dress shoe.

*My right foot is 1/2 size larger than my left.